Law,
Psychiatry,
and
Morality

Law,
Psychiatry,
and
Morality

ESSAYS AND ANALYSIS

by Alan A. Stone, M.D.

*Touroff-Glueck Professor
of Law and Psychiatry
Harvard University*

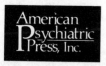

American
Psychiatric
Press, Inc.

1400 K STREET, N.W.
WASHINGTON, D.C. 20005

Cover design by Sam Haltom
Text design by Tim Clancy and Richard E. Farkas
Typeset by Unicorn Graphics
Printed by R. R. Donnelley & Sons Co.

Library of Congress Cataloging in Publication Data
Stone, Alan A.
Law, psychiatry, and morality.
Includes bibliographical references.
1. Insanity—Jurisprudence—United States—Addresses,
essays, lectures. 2. Forensic psychiatry—United
States—Addresses, essays, lectures. 3. Psychiatrists—
Legal status, laws, etc.—United States—Addresses, essays,
lectures. 4. Psychiatric ethics—Addresses, essays,
lectures. I. Title.
KF9242.A5S76 1984   614'.1   84-3000
ISBN 0-88048-028-9
ISBN 0-88048-038-6 (pbk.)
ISBN 0-88048-209-5 (trade pbk.)

for my mother and father

Contents

Preface

These essays are attempts to think through some of the major problems in law and psychiatry as I now understand them. My understanding has been shaped by my personal and intellectual experiences, some of which I would like to share with the reader. In particular, I want to explain why questions of morality now seem so important to me in thinking about psychiatry and its relationship to law.

I began my career as a psychoanalytic psychiatrist at McLean Hospital interested in the treatment of very sick patients. Longitudinal study of child development was my first research interest, because it seemed particularly pertinent both to the continuing scientific development of psychoanalytic theory and to the understanding of regressed psychotic behavior.

I was quite naive about law when Professor Alan Dershowitz invited me to Harvard Law School in 1965 to teach with him a seminar on psychoanalytic theory and legal assumptions based on the Katz, Goldstein, and Dershowitz casebook, *Psychoanalysis, Psychiatry and Law*. The seminar was well received by the students and the collaboration was intellectually rewarding. Alan Dershowitz asked me to join him in teaching a course on psychiatry and law. Thus my career unexpectedly took a different direction than I had imagined. In 1968 the Law School secured a grant from the National Institute of Mental Health which allowed me to spend an academic year in legal studies. The transplant took and I became a member of the Law Faculty.

During our years of teaching the course on Psychoanalytic Theory and Legal Assumptions, Alan Dershowitz became convinced that psychoanalysis had rather little of practical value to offer law. He turned his interests to other matters, and I continued this course on my own. I had come to this teaching as someone versed in psychoanalytic theory and not in law. And as I now think back on those days, I realize that I then believed that psychoanalysis was a discipline separate from morality.

Law, I assumed, combined certain psychological assumptions with

morality, legal doctrine, politics, history, etcetera. Thus, I then thought
that the task was to tease out the law's psychological assumptions and
examine them in the light of psychoanalytic theory. I now believe this
was a basic misunderstanding on my part.

Paradoxically, I had always believed that psychiatry and psychoanalysis stood halfway between the sciences and the humanities.
Indeed, it was this posture of the profession which originally attracted
me (and I believe many of my contemporaries as well) to it. But by some
strange mental gymnastics, I assumed that morality was not part of the
mixture—this was a blind spot I now attribute to my adherence to
Freud as he had been understood in the United States, that is, with
psychoanalytic ego psychology built on.

Freud's psychoanalysis was among other things a revolutionary
criticism of the dominant morality of his time. But ego psychology,
particularly in America, emphasized adaptation, ego and superego
development, and other "scientific" concepts. By so doing it made
psychoanalytic psychiatry seem to be less a revolutionary criticism and
more a part of "ordinary science." The person and the self, central to
any moral theory, were decomposed into objectified structures and
functions. All of this now seems wrong to me, not just as a matter of abstract theory, but as a matter of the most practical importance for
psychiatry as well as psychoanalysis. It seems to me that in their own
ways Roy Schafer, Heinz Kohut, Karen Horney, and Erik Erikson have
all been struggling with this same problem—reconstructing the self.
This task is essential if one is to get beyond the untenable position that
psychoanalysis or psychiatry are morally neutral. In fact, I believe, it is
essential for any coherent theory of the human experience.

Teaching law and psychiatry with Alan Dershowitz, a collaboration which has continued over the last fifteen years, gave me two great
advantages. He introduced me to powerful civil libertarian arguments
against every element of discretionary authority that the law granted to
psychiatry, without denying the reality of mental illness. This education
in law and psychiatry from a civil libertarian point of view came just at
the time when that approach took on enormous importance in the
courts. Out of my dialogue with Alan Dershowitz, I was able to develop
my own positions, tested against his argument. Thus I was prepared and
able to play a part in psychiatry's response to legal reform and had the
opportunity to be involved in direct ways in many of the major landmark
cases.

During my recent years at Harvard Law School, other colleagues have influenced my thinking in important ways. Roberto Unger's work on the theory of the self and the passions has been very important to the development of my own thinking. Duncan Kennedy and I read together over several years Hegel's *Phenomenology of Spirit* and Sartre's *Being and Nothingness*. Duncan made much understandable that would have otherwise been incomprehensible in the "Unity of Spirit," "The Master and Slave," "The Reef of Solipsism," and "The Look." He is an unrelenting critic of received wisdom and at the same time a gifted psychologist.

Sartre's existential psychoanalysis has had a considerable influence on my ideas. The unconscious and bad faith are now strange bedfellows in my mind, contradictory but somehow both necessary to understanding the human condition.

Several of my former students have become colleagues and teachers, but I believe they consider me a difficult student. Among the lawyers are Joel Klein, Clifford Stromberg, Stephen Morse, and Michael Moore. Among the psychiatrists are Loren Roth and Paul Appelbaum.

During most of my years as a Harvard Law Professor I have had student research assistants. All of them have helped me in important ways, particularly in my legal research. My most recent research assistants, who assisted with this book, have been Stephanie Martin Glennon, a second year Harvard law student who took on the laboring oar, and her classmate Claire Gutterman, who helped at the finish.

John Hodson, formerly a philosophy professor and now a third year Harvard law student, worked with me over the summer of 1983. David Zatzkis, a recent graduate and now an attorney in Los Angeles, pitched in and was particularly helpful with the final drafts of my essay on Psychiatry and the Supreme Court.

My wife Sue Smart Stone, who is herself an attorney, was my principal legal research assistant in the two essays that deal with malpractice. She has always listened to the first draft of everything. She is my original reader. My son David Stone, a third year Harvard law student, helped me with the essay on Psychiatry and Violence. His own work on prosecutorial strategies is cited there.

My son Douglas Stone, a physicist who is also trained in philosophy, helped me to reason through the essays on psychiatry and morality. It is a great good fortune to have a son who can help you order your most ambitious thoughts. My daughter Karen Stone, a psychologist, is the only member of the family who has not worked on this book. But she is busy doing her own research in child development, and I therefore feel she has taken over the original family business.

My secretary, Kathleen Harrison, has helped me over a number of crisis points, and she has patiently translated my difficult longhand into the endless drafts that went to the word-processing machine. She has been an essential link in the chain of this book's coming into being. As for Joette Chancy-Borden and Deborah Gallagher, who operate Harvard Law School's word processor, I am greatly in their debt.

During one year while I worked on parts of this book, I was supported at the Center for Advanced Study in the Behavioral Sciences, by the John D. and Catherine T. MacArthur Foundation, and by the Commonwealth Fund. The latter also supported my first book, *Longitudinal Studies of Child Behavior*. I am, therefore, twice grateful to them. My interest in and experiences with the international problems of political misuse of psychiatry was supported by a Guggenheim Fellowship. I am most appreciative of the enthusiastic cooperation I have gotten from Ronald McMillen and the editors of the American Psychiatric Press. There is no better remedy for an author's doldrums than a receptive editor.

Harvard Law School has supported all of my work for many years. It is an extraordinary, exciting, and stimulating intellectual environment. I find it hard to believe that I could have found a better place in which to grow intellectually. These essays are intended to be provocative and to stir the reader, who should feel entitled to disagree. They are the result of years of dialogue with students, who, it is my hope, felt challenged to think some more. I hope the reader will have the same experience.

Alan A. Stone, M.D.

Acknowledgments

"Psychiatry and Violence" was presented as the Edwin Lipinski Distinguished Lecture at the Annual Meeting of the Canadian Psychiatric Association in 1983.

"The Ethics of Forensic Psychiatry: A View from the Ivory Tower" was first presented as an invited lecture to the American Academy of Psychiatry and the Law. A shortened version with responses appears in *The Bulletin of the American Academy of Psychiatry and the Law* (Vol. 5, pp. 209–219, 1984).

"The Trial of John Hinckley" was an invited special lecture to the American Psychiatric Association at its Annual Meeting in 1983. I am grateful to them for obtaining for my use the transcript of the psychiatric testimony.

"Psychiatry and the Supreme Court" was given as the Isaac Ray Award Lecture at UCLA Medical School.

"Psychiatric Abuse and Legal Reform: Two Ways to Make a Bad Situation Worse" was presented at the University of Virginia as the First Memorial Lecture for Browning Hoffman. It was published in the *International Journal of Law and Psychiatry* (Vol. 5, pp. 9–28, 1982 [Copyright 1982 by Pergamon Press, Ltd. Reprinted in revised form with permission.]) This essay has been updated to include comments on recently decided cases involving the right to refuse treatment.

Two of these essays are updated, expanded, and reworked versions of previously published papers. "The *Tarasoff* Case and Some of Its Progeny: Suing Psychotherapists to Safeguard Society" is based on an article published in the *Harvard Law Review* (Vol. 90, No. 2, December 1976 [Copyright 1976 by the Harvard Law Review Association. Reprinted in revised form with permission.]). "Sexual Exploitation of Patients in Psychotherapy" combines and amplifies two papers published in the *American Journal of Psychiatry* (Vol. 133, No. 10, pp. 1138–1114, 1976 [Copyright 1976 by the American Psychiatric Association]; Vol. 140, No. 2, pp. 195–197, 1983 [Copyright 1983 by the American Psychiatric Association]; both reprinted in revised form with permission).

"Psychiatry and Morality: Three Criticisms" and "Psychiatry as Morality" were presented as the Tanner Lectures on Human Values at Stanford University on March 31 and April 5, 1982. The lectures were published by the University of Utah Press and Cambridge University Press (Copyright 1983 by The Tanner Lectures on Human Values, Inc. Reprinted in revised form with permission.) and have been minimally altered.

"Morality for Psychiatry" is based on my Presidential Address to the American Psychiatric Association, which was originally published in the *American Journal of Psychiatry*, Vol. 137, No. 8, pp. 887–893, 1980 (Copyright 1980 by the American Psychiatric Association. Reprinted in revised form with permission.). With a new introduction and some alterations, it has become the last essay in this collection.

Law,
Psychiatry,
and
Morality

I

Political Misuse of Psychiatry:
A Tale of Two Generals

A REMARKABLE HISTORICAL COINCIDENCE occurred between the two great world powers during the first years of the decade of the 1960s. Senior army generals in both the Soviet Union and the United States were charged with crimes against their state. Both claimed to be true patriots, and risked their military careers by criticizing their governments. Both aired their views in a dramatic fashion—the Soviet general at a Communist party meeting, the American general in Congressional hearings. Both in the Soviet Union and in the United States, government lawyers high in the political hierarchy impugned the sanity of the generals and thus effectively discredited their political activities. And in both cases, distinguished psychiatrists cooperated in that process.

The Soviet general, Petro Grigorenko, claimed to be a true Leninist. He attacked the Soviet regime for allowing Khrushchev and the "cult of personality" to interfere with the withering away of the state. The American general, Edwin Walker, claimed to be a true American. He attacked Presidents Eisenhower and Kennedy for violating the principles of American democracy by imposing racial integration and by being "soft" on Communism. He claimed to be a true Jeffersonian

3

American. Both generals, after being admonished for criticizing their "corrupt" governments—and both eventually forced out of the military—went on to participate in what they thought were courageous acts of civil disobedience.

In both countries, psychiatrists diagnosed their unwilling patients as paranoid and raised questions about their competency to stand trial and their responsibility for their alleged crimes against the state. Both generals considered the diagnosis of paranoia an affront to their integrity and dignity. There was criticism of the psychiatrists who participated in both cases, and there were claims of political misuse of psychiatry in both countries.

Here, however, the parallels end; the fates of the two generals diverge. These parallels and divergences tell a story about law and psychiatry in the two countries—a story relevant to the international claims and counterclaims of political misuse of psychiatry. These claims, particularly those against the Soviet Union, have torn apart the World Psychiatric Association and put an end to psychiatry's detente.

J. K. Wing, a British psychiatrist, hoped to avert this result. He wrote in 1974:

> Complaints of *malpractice* have been made about medical services in several parts of the world, notably the United States and the Soviet Union, but our country has not been immune from criticism [emphasis added].[1]

The term "malpractice" was obviously carefully chosen, given the tone of Wing's article. It was meant to depoliticize the international charges and the countercharges and to medicalize them. History took a different direction than Wing had hoped. The All-Union Soviet Society of neuropathologists and psychiatrists was condemned in 1977. The World Psychiatric Association undertook efforts to investigate allegations of ethical abuses around the world. By 1983 the Soviet Union and a number of other nations responded by resigning from the Association. As in the case with the two generals, in reality the problem was not "malpractice" in the usual sense of that word. Consider the Soviet situation. General Grigorenko has not claimed that his psychiatrists were medically negligent. He insisted that they colluded with the K.G.B. and with Khrushchev to discredit him, his criticisms, and his dissident activities. The Soviet psychiatrist, Semyon Gluzman, who was himself imprisoned, had reported that Soviet psychiatrists were intentionally and duplicitously misdiagnosing, confining, and abusing Soviet dissidents with unnecessary treatment. General Grigorenko was

Gluzman's chief example.[2] Similar claims were made by many others, and these claims were widely credited in the West, leading to the condemnation of Soviet psychiatrists not for malpractice or negligence, but for intentional willful political misuse of psychiatry against dissidents.

THE CASE FOR SOVIET PSYCHIATRY

There have been some within the Western psychiatric establishment who disagree with this condemnation. Since political condemnation has prevailed and the accusations against the Soviet Union have been much publicized,[3] it may be useful to suggest the kind of arguments that dissenters from that condemnation might make. Their basic claim is that the problem cannot be laid at the door of Soviet psychiatry. Rather, it is the Soviet law and the Soviet regime which bear the responsibility. The Soviet legal system does not allow for the freedom of dissent which Anglo-American standards permit. Soviet dissidents who criticize the state face possible legal sanctions under Articles 70, 72, 142, 190.1, and 227 of the Soviet Criminal Code.[4] There are complex and debatable legal questions about these "crimes." Lawyers for the dissidents interpret Soviet law as requiring that criticisms of the state must be false and intended to slander the state in order to be criminal. They have also challenged the legality of the trial procedures applied to dissidents. But if these are debatable legal questions, it is undebatable that under Soviet law the Presidium is the ultimate legal authority. Andropov, Brezhnev, Khrushchev: these men make the decisions.

Whether or not these laws as interpreted by the Soviet regime and its courts are just, when they are violated, Soviet authorities can be expected to arrest and prosecute violators. One may object to the laws themselves or to the selective enforcement of them by a harsh regime, but to condemn the Soviet courts for failing to apply American constitutional law is simply an exercise in parochialism. Although arguments have been made to the contrary, it would be fair to say that many Soviet dissidents have knowingly engaged in acts of civil disobedience. They have challenged the established legal order.

A second problem follows from this. When a Soviet dissident like Anatoly Koryagin, the consulting psychiatrist to the *Moscow Working Commission to Investigate the Use of Psychiatry for Political Purposes*, was arrested and charged with a crime, it could not be dismissed as a trumped-up charge.

One cannot assume that the court that convicted him of "anti-Soviet agitation and propaganda" was engaging in conscious and cynical duplicity. Koryagin wrote in *The Lancet* of April 11, 1981:

> All the people I examined had joined the ranks of the mentally ill because they did or said things which in our country are considered anti-Soviet.[5]

The author was by existing Soviet standards committing a crime. Koryagin's report may have been truthful, but it is not hard to understand that a Soviet court would determine that it was not truthful, and that his article was written for the purpose "of subverting or weakening the Soviet regime." It may be true, as Western lawyers claimed, that under Soviet law Doctor Koryagin should have been entitled to call witnesses to prove the truthfulness of his claims. This would have allowed him to turn his trial into a trial of the regime's political misuse of psychiatry. It is not surprising that the court refused. Unlike the "patients" he described, Doctor Koryagin was charged with a crime and convicted, rather than pronounced mentally ill. Reports are that he is being treated very harshly in prison and has been subjected to physical beatings. Indeed, his fate is typical of what has befallen the *Moscow Working Commission* (e.g., V. Bakhmin, A. Podrabinek, F. Serebrov, L. Ternovsky, I. Grivnina).[6]

The upshot of these arguments is that Soviet dissidents, under Soviet law as interpreted by the current regime, can be sent to prisons, to labor camps, or to mental hospitals. Thus, defenders of Soviet psychiatry claim that what the West called psychiatric *terrorism* may in fact have been psychiatric *humanity*, diverting dissidents to the least punitive alternative.[7] Wing suggested this possibility in 1974:

> The Soviet doctor claims that he is acting humanely and that in essence, the part he plays is not different from that of the American psychiatrists who saved Ezra Pound from execution.[8]

Along these lines, an anonymous Soviet writer has claimed that,

> even the notorious Lunts [a Soviet psychiatrist alleged to have been an officer of the K.G.B.], who died prematurely, affirmed in confidential conversations that, when he was snatching victims from the grasp of the K.G.B. and found them [not guilty by reason of insanity], it was only out of good intentions that he sometimes "laid it on a bit thick."[9]

More will be said about Doctor Lunts, who sat on a panel of experts that declared General Grigorenko insane. But it should be noted that if even Lunts can be excused, then the case for condemning Soviet psychiatrists is very much weakened, because in many allegations he (along with Professor Georgy Morozov) was a central figure. General Grigorenko maintains that he saw Lunts wearing a K.G.B. uniform.[10]

The anonymous Soviet author who makes excuses for Lunts continues:

> So, is there psychiatric terrorism in the U.S.S.R. or isn't there? There is. And who practices it? Government Agencies [the K.G.B. and the courts]. In the practice of this terrorism, the psychiatrists are used as a benighted mass—people who know not what they do. Because of this there should be a shift of emphasis in the international protest against psychiatric terrorism. It is senseless to accuse the psychiatrists of deliberately distorting diagnoses to suit the purposes of the K.G.B., because this does not happen—with perhaps a negligible number of easily exposed exceptions.
>
> What does exist is the barbaric practice of confining "political" patients in special [prison] psychiatric hospitals. In the name of justice, and to the shame of the psychiatrists, it must be said that following the successful example of the Serbsky Institute, they do not object to including in their expert findings recommendations that "politicals" who are mentally incompetent but not socially dangerous be confined for compulsory treatment. But where and when have there not been overly-zealous lackeys of the State system?[11]

Dr. Abraham Halpern has pressed the defense of Soviet psychia-trists even further. The problem in his view is not the K.G.B. or the So-viet Regime but the insanity defense and the "evils which follow it like a shadow in every country where the rule is employed." Halpern, an American psychiatrist, declared on the English language service of Moscow radio that the Soviet All-Union Society of Neuropathologists and Psychiatrists had been "defamed in such a scurrilous and vilifying way [that it] shames the whole world of psychiatry."[12] Explaining his remarks subsequently, he noted that he had pointed his finger at the Soviet legal system and "the exculpatory insanity defense."[13]

THE CASE AGAINST SOVIET PSYCHIATRY

The anonymous Soviet writer who condemns his state while defending Soviet psychiatrists nonetheless admits a specific psychiatric abuse: confining mentally incompetent dissidents in institutions for the crimi-nally insane. Reviewing the many claims of Soviet misuse of psychiatry over the past 15 years, this admission emerges as the most indisputable indictment.

The Soviet Union's mental health laws, as written, are in fact quite progressive[14]—particularly in regard to persons charged with crimes. Under Soviet law, a person whose competence and criminal responsibility are in question can be evaluated as an outpatient in an ordinary mental hospital or in a special facility for those deemed "socially dangerous."[15] None of the prominent Soviet dissidents engaged in acts of violence. Yet many, including General Grigorenko, were confined in "special facilities." Even if, despite all the damning evidence to the contrary, Soviet psychiatrists had in good faith diagnosed all of these dissidents as mentally ill, how could they in good faith have found them "socially dangerous"? I put this question to the Dean of Soviet Psychiatry, A. Snezhnevsky, at a meeting in his hospital in Moscow in 1978. His answer was instructive in many ways.

First, he pointed out that this was not the criticism made by Western psychiatrists when they had condemned the Soviet All-Union Society. The condemnation had been a broadside attack, not a specific indictment. Second, he emphasized that from the Russian perspective, the West was viewed as having tried for more than half a century to destroy the "Revolution." Therefore, attacks on the "Revolution"—that is, dissident political activities—were in the Soviet perspective *socially* dangerous. Finally, he relied on the same argument relied on by American forensic psychiatrists who are challenged about their role in the courts. They assert, as did Snezhnevsky, that the ultimate responsibility is not the psychiatrist's, but the judge's. Psychiatrists testify; courts decide. Snezhnevsky also intimated that psychiatrists know in these cases that the court will decide on a special facility, and there is thus little point in suggesting a different disposition.

Western criticism of Soviet psychiatry has also focused on Snezhnevsky personally, not only because he sat on the original commission which declared Grigorenko insane and recommended that he be sent to a special institute, but also because he is principally responsible for the Soviet concept of schizophrenia, which encompasses a "sluggish type" manifest by "reformerism" among other symptoms. This diagnostic scheme can readily be applied to dissidents. The Soviet diagnosis of schizophrenia is clearly much broader than is the definition in the West, and includes types of disorders which Western psychiatrists would diagnose as character disorders—including schizoid, schizotypal, and narcissistic disorders.

But there is, in my opinion, no evidence that the Snezhnevsky nosology was designed to reach dissidents. Soviet psychiatry as influenced by Snezhnevsky's nosology is very much rooted in the

Kraepelinian era, with its biological orientation. As is now the case in the West, there is in the Soviet Union a strong presumption that schizophrenia is a biological if not a genetic disorder. Distinguished Western psychiatrists have suggested that schizophrenia and the "schizoidia" (schizotypal, schizoid, narcissistic, paranoid personality disorders) are one genetic disorder.[16] Snezhnevsky, in much the same vein, has taken a further step, and has included the schizoidia as sluggish forms of schizophrenia in his definition.

The most divergent aspect of the Soviet classification, from a Western perspective, is the assumption that involutional and senile changes are associated with the emergence of schizophrenic disorder. Soviet psychiatrists identify schizophrenic disorder where Western psychiatrists would find involutional melancholia. Schizophrenia in the Soviet Union is not a diagnosis limited to disorders which begin before middle age.[17] However, it should be noted that in DSM-III involutional melancholia has become either major depression *or paranoid disorder*. Thus Soviet and American nosology have much in common. Nonetheless, given this broad and encompassing concept of schizophrenia and given the rather common assumption by psychiatrists that schizophrenics are not criminally responsible, it is not hard to understand how Soviet psychiatrists might determine that dissidents are incompetent and insane.

Wing put the issue very well. Under Western eyes the problem is:

Should a person who is not severely mentally ill by our standards be regarded as [not] responsible for an action which we would not regard as a crime?[18]

Under Soviet eyes the problem becomes:

Is a person who is suffering from a slowly developing form of schizophrenia [not] responsible for an action which is likely to land him at the very least, in a labor camp for three years?[19]

Supporters of Soviet Union psychiatrists can add still other excuses. Psychiatry in the Soviet Union is highly bureaucratized, and there is less room for independent judgment than there is in the West. The Soviet psychiatric bureaucracy, like all bureaucracies, must be responsive to political pressure from above. Furthermore, the psychiatrists themselves would risk a great deal if they were to depart from the party line. It is an act of courage simply to remain silent, and it takes more than courage to contradict those in the psychiatric hierarchy who are part of the political power structure. Indeed the fate of Dr. Semyon Gluzman and Dr. Anatoly Koryagin is evidence for these contentions.

These added considerations are relevant to the attempts of the World Psychiatric Association to require Soviet Union psychiatrists to investi' gate and report allegations of political misuse. The argument is that the psychiatrists who might attempt to comply with these requests would themselves be risking a great deal. Nor could they acknowledge those risks to the World Psychiatric Association without risk. (There are of course contradictory views.)

Perhaps the most convincing evidence for all of these arguments can be found by examining treatment of Soviet dissidents since the Western condemnation of Soviet misuse of psychiatry. Like the Mos' cow group, these dissidents have been given Soviet justice without benefit of Soviet psychiatry. They have been sentenced to harsh labor camps and to prisons.[20] But even the anonymous writer from the Soviet Union acknowledges "a negligible number of easily exposed exceptions" and in addition underscores the culpability of Soviet psychiatrists involved in confining harmless incompetent dissidents with the socially dangerous criminally insane. General Grigorenko claimed his treatment was an example of both these practices.

GENERAL GRIGORENKO

General Grigorenko makes a very good test case as to whether there has been political abuse of psychiatry in the Soviet Union.[21] A prominent figure in the Soviet Army and in the Communist Party, he criticized the regime, allied himself with dissident groups, and was charged with a crime. He was found mentally ill (paranoid) and not responsible, and was confined for long periods in various psychiatric facilities, including "special" institutions for the criminally insane.

When I was in Moscow and met with Professor Snezhnevsky, General Grigorenko, who had come to the United States, had already requested that I examine him. I asked Professor Snezhnevsky how he would feel about such an examination. Without hesitation, he urged that the examination take place. He had himself examined General Grigorenko and asserted that an objective examination would prove that his diagnosis of chronic paranoia had been correct and that Grigorenko was still paranoid. The confidence of his assertion should not be ignored. It should also not be ignored that Snezhnevsky and the other Soviet psychiatrists claimed that Grigorenko was paranoid by Kraepelinian standards and not by diagnostic criteria unique to the

Soviet Union. Thus, this is not a case in which one needs to worry about divergent diagnostic concepts.

It may be appropriate to add here something of my personal impression of Snezhnevsky. He was bright, candid, and engaging, and even through a translator the conversation had a sparkle. He was certainly in sharp contrast to the guarded, cautious psychiatric bureau-crats one meets in the Soviet Union and elsewhere. His personality had not become submerged in his role; he did not seem to be looking over his shoulder or repeating vacuous verbiage. Of course, he had a prominent and secure position in Soviet psychiatry and the Soviet power struc-ture.

There is another reason why General Grigorenko is a particularly good test case. Many of the Soviet dissidents are Jews, and their criticism of the regime, if it is not deemed a manifestation of mental illness, is often attributed to Zionist or cosmopolitan ideology, which are also deemed anti-Soviet. Thus, discussions of political or psychiatric abuse of dissidents in the Soviet Union frequently involve the Jewish question—with explicit or implicit allegations of Soviet anti-Semitism and all of the attendant emotions aroused by memories of centuries of pogroms and persecution in Russia. We are spared those complications in considering General Grigorenko. He is Ukrainian by birth and was raised in the Orthodox church until he left it to join the Communist Party.

Grigorenko was diagnosed at least three times by Soviet psychia-trists sitting as legally constituted commissions to inquire into his sanity—in April 1964, August 1969, and November 1969.[22] The commission is the Soviet legal system's inquisitional alternative to our adversarial psychiatric testimony. General Grigorenko's lawyer was not permitted to select psychiatrists to give independent testimony. The first commission, which included both the late Professor Lunts and Snezhnevsky, diagnosed Grigorenko as suffering from mental illness in the form of a paranoid delusional development of his personality, accompanied by early signs of cerebral arteriosclerosis. Doctor Lunts, reporting later on that diagnosis, said that the symptoms of paranoid development were "reformist ideas" and "an overestimation of his own personality reaching messianic proportions." Grigorenko was also said to be "emotionally caught up in his own experiences and unshakably convinced of the rightness of his actions." Other symptoms included "unhealthy suspiciousness" and "emotional excitability."

A second commission, meeting some four years later in Tashkent and chaired by Doctor Detengof, could find none of the symptoms or manifestations cited by the Lunts commission. Its diagnosis and evalua-tion was that

> Grigorenko's [criminal] activity had a purposeful character, it was related to concrete events and facts . . . .It did not reveal any signs of illness or delusions.[23]

Doctor Detengof's commission noted the 1964 Serbsky diagnosis, but stated that they could find no evidence that the conditions cited earlier had continued or recurred. This is an important episode for two reasons. First, it indicates that psychiatrists in the Soviet Union are not part of a monolithic apparatus that always produces the same result. Second, it means that Soviet psychiatrists who understand the social and cultural context of Russia did not diagnose Grigorenko's dissident ideas as paranoia. Yet, three months later, having been brought back from Tashkent to a Moscow prison, Grigorenko was again diagnosed as paranoid. The commission, chaired by Doctor G. Morozov and includ-ing Doctor Lunts among its members, recommended his return to a special psychiatric facility for the socially dangerous.

It was ten years later when General Grigorenko asked to be examined in the West. (How he came to be in the United States will be described below.) At the time of his original request, he intended to return to the Soviet Union to continue his dissident activities. By the time I had returned from my visit to the Soviet Union, Grigorenko's Soviet citizenship had been revoked. As Grigorenko later wrote in his memoirs, the Soviet Union had twice punished him while saying that he was not responsible for his behavior. Yet, if his criticism of the Soviet Union was based in paranoia, then he should not have been deprived of his general's pension and his citizenship. He had received the worst of both the world of law and the world of psychiatry.

Grigorenko nonetheless still wanted to undertake a thorough psychiatric examination. He hoped to prove his sanity. Furthermore, he was prepared to waive in advance all privilege of confidentiality. A rigorous evaluation was set up for him both in Boston and New York. In Boston he underwent neurological, psychological, neuropsychological, and psychiatric examinations.

Unfortunately, General Walker never requested such an examina-tion, and consequently it is not possible to compare the men on that basis. Therefore, it would be helpful first to present Grigorenko's political, military, and legal history in a way that is comparable with what is known of General Walker from public records. I shall then describe Grigorenko's psychiatric history as it emerged during the course of my personal examination.

General Petro Grigoryevich Grigorenko[24] was born in 1907 in the Ukraine. He became an ardent communist at an early age and served in the Soviet Union's military ranks for more than thirty years. His combat career began in 1939 in Mongolia, and after World War II he worked for sixteen years in the Frunze Military Academy in Moscow, where he served as a specialist in cybernetics research. General Grigorenko accumulated many military accolades and promotions for the service he gave to his country, and was active in the Communist Party as well.

The first public display of Grigorenko's shift from the official party line came in 1961. This incident came after the famous 20th Party Congress at which Nikita Khrushchev had for the first time publicly criticized Stalin. Grigorenko made a speech at a Party Congress, criticizing what he saw as the post-Stalin subversion of Leninist principles. He warned against the continuing political corruption and the danger to the Revolution created by the Cult of Personality. Implicitly he criticized Khrushchev for continuing the corruption and the Cult of Personality, which prevented the "withering away of the State." His party delegation from the Frunze Military Academy deemed his speech "politically immature" and sought to deprive him of his delegate's credentials.[25] Eventually the party elite blamed Grigorenko for "distortion of the party line on the question of the personality cult."[26]

In an oddly prophetic moment shortly thereafter, a friend told Grigorenko that the "only thing that [could have saved him was] a diagnosis by a psychiatrist that [he] did not know what [he] was saying."[27] The repercussions of this speech by Grigorenko, and its impact upon his reputation among the ruling elite, were dramatic. He was not immediately considered *persona non grata* or removed from military service, but was sent off to the Far East in January 1962. There he headed the Operations Branch of the Fifth Army—a position specially designated to diminish his powers.[28]

Grigorenko did not cease to vocalize his opinions about the official party line with respect to Leninist doctrine. In 1963 he and his son Gregory, then a student at the Artillery Engineering Academy, organized the "Alliance for Struggle for Rebirth of Leninism."[29] Their primary tool of instruction was leaflets, which soon came to the attention of the Soviet hierarchy. Grigorenko was arrested in 1963 for carrying "anti-Soviet materials."[30]

Rather than sentencing him on the charges which led to his arrest, the authorities ordered Grigorenko to be committed to the Serbsky

Scientific Research Institution for Forensic Psychiatry in order to undergo psychiatric examination and evaluation. In his memoirs, General Grigorenko reports that the pretext for his commitment was a report of "traumatic cerebropathy" (an episode of shell shock[31]) contained in his medical records. A number of other minor ailments were also considered relevant premonitory symptoms of his condition.

Grigorenko's report of the ensuing psychiatric interrogation is ironic, particularly when considered in the context of his later conflicts with Soviet authorities:

> All my replies were evaluated as the judgments of an abnormal person. She [the psychiatrist] also could not understand historical analogies, and she evaluated them only in psychiatric terms. If I referred to Chernyshevsky she would write: 'He compares himself to Chernyshevsky.' If I referred to Lenin she would write: 'He compares himself to Lenin.'[32]

In a critical portion of the interrogation, Grigorenko responded to the psychiatrist's questions about his attitude toward Nikita Khrushchev. The General said that Khrushchev was a "zero" who would "not remain in power long" and would "be out by this autumn."[33] Soon after this examination, in April 1964, a commission of experts determined that Grigorenko was insane,[34] noting specifically the supposed delusional grandiosity inherent in his prophecy about Khrushchev, and he was sent to Lefortoro prison to await trial. Because he had been diagnosed mentally ill, he was not allowed to attend the trial at which the court found him not responsible. He was transferred to the Leningrad Special Psychiatric Hospital. But then, ironically, his "prophecy" came true. Khrushchev was in fact removed from office in October—unfortunately for Grigorenko and his family, not before Khrushchev had insisted on demoting him to a private and depriving him of his pension despite his supposed insanity.

Ordinarily, persons in the Soviet Union who have been found insane must undergo six months of psychiatric treatment before being granted a new hearing. But in 1965 the post-Khruschev government, in a highly unusual move, approved his wife's application to annul the General's diagnosis and compulsory psychiatric treatment.[35] Grigorenko was freed.

The former General had to seek work as a porter and had little energy for anything else. But by 1966 Grigorenko's further activities had led him deep into the human rights movement. Soon he was at the heart of the activist group containing the Soviet Union's most vocal political dissidents. He became involved in causes like The Alliance for Liberation of the Ukraine and the Ukrainian Rebel Army. He opposed the Soviet occupation of Czechoslovakia in 1968. And he became an advocate on behalf of the Crimean Tatars who had been deported to Central Asia, the Urals, and Kazakstan by the terms of Stalin's decree. Nearly half of the Crimean Tatars allegedly had perished during the relocation.[36]

In 1969 Grigorenko went to Tashkent and was arrested there because of his activities on behalf of the Crimean Tatars. Again he was forced to submit to psychiatric evaluation of his sanity. The General later explained his perception of the government's actions:

> The people in power did not want to create a precedent of a general who was seditious, a precedent of a general who was critical of the power, so a decision was made to declare me mentally ill, to make a pa-tient out of me.[37]

As we shall see, General Walker had the same impression of the people in power in the United States.

But a panel of Tashkent psychiatrists declared Grigorenko sane. This meant the government would have to press criminal charges. A public trial involving General Grigorenko was not without problems. It would certainly have had the potential to create a public event for all So-viet dissidents, and would have brought world-wide attention to the plight of the Crimean Tatars. The government opted to bring Grigorenko back to Moscow, where Professor Lunts and a new commis-sion again declared Grigorenko insane and again committed him to a special psychiatric hospital.[38] As in the United States, a "sentence" of psychiatric treatment after being found not guilty by reason of insanity has infinitely expansive capacities, and may be used to justify incarcera-tion for a far longer period of time than was statutorily authorized as punishment for the crimes alleged.[39]

Grigorenko was to spend more than five years undergoing involun-tary confinement in Soviet psychiatric hospitals, most of that time in virtual solitary confinement in an institution for the criminally insane. It was, finally, concerted political pressure from outside the Soviet Union that effected Grigorenko's release from psychiatric confinement. Water-gate was closing in on President Nixon, but he made plans to visit Moscow. Alexander Solzhenitsyn, already in the United States, con-tacted Nixon and asked him to appeal on Grigorenko's behalf.[40] In 1974, just a day before Nixon's visit to Moscow, Grigorenko was released.

Shortly thereafter, he, his wife, and one of their sons were able to

secure visas for a trip to the United States, where General Grigorenko
was scheduled to undergo a prostate operation. He resolved to behave in
such a way that the Soviet government would have no excuse to
terminate his citizenship during his absence, but in February 1978 his
citizenship was revoked. The reason given was that Grigorenko had
been "systematically carrying out actions which are incompatible with
citizenship in the U.S.S.R. By his conduct he is doing harm to the
prestige of the U.S.S.R."[41] Grigorenko, who began as a peasant in the
Ukraine and rose to the rank of General in the Soviet Army, had become
a refugee in the United States.

The American Psychiatric Examination

On a cold day in December 1978, General Grigorenko came to my
office at Harvard Law School in Cambridge, Massachusetts. He was
accompanied by Boris Zoubok, a Soviet-trained psychiatrist who had
emigrated to the West and who would serve as his translator. The
General spoke no English. I had my own translator, since it seemed to
me the best way to ensure the reliability of the translation. The general
was tall, solid, military in his bearing, and striking in appearance because
he had completely shaved his balding head. He was in his seventies and
looked his age. His gait was slow and his feet were wide based. The four
of us first went to lunch in the Law School Faculty Dining Room. I
wanted to observe the General in an informal setting.

The General dined with dignity and served himself from the buffet
with an apparent eye for balanced nutrition. Conversation was not easy,
and Grigorenko must have been aware that I was watching every move
he made. We then went to a room which had been arranged so that I
could tape the psychiatric examination. Professor Snezhnevsky had said
that Grigorenko had been and was still paranoid. The questions I had
posed to myself were these: Was Grigorenko now paranoid? Did he have
fixed ideas? Would he react in a stubborn, hostile, persecuted, or
grandiose way when his ideas were challenged? Would I find evidence
of denial and projection? Would the General claim that his psychiatrists
had abused him? If so, in what ways? Finally, there was the question
whether, even if Grigorenko was not paranoid now, one could say that
he had not been paranoid in the past.

Psychiatrists have good reason to be concerned about their
countertransference, and here was a situation ready made for
countertransference. First, I was President-elect of the American Psychiatric Association at the time, and even though I was not examining

Grigorenko in that capacity, I had no doubt that it played a part in my selection as an examiner and would have significance in the future for him and for me. Second, I realized that my experience with generals, even American generals, was rather limited. What, I wondered, was appropriate rigidity, pomposity, and narcissism for a general? The closest equivalent I had was college presidents and deans. Third, I was worried about the ethics of what I was doing. Grigorenko had put his trust in me to do an objective examination. So had Doctor Snezhnevsky. I was sitting in judgment on Grigorenko and on Soviet psychiatrists. I knew that I could not please them both. But what if I found Grigorenko was paranoid? Could I ethically *publish* a report to that effect relying on his prior consent? He had himself written in his memoirs:

> This is my confession. I have honestly attempted to tell the truth the way I see it. But why should I confess in public? It is because my life has outgrown the bounds of ordinariness and become a social phenom-enon.

But his memoirs were written as a defense of his personal integrity. They clearly tell his side of the story. He controlled the content of his autobiography, but he could not control or even know in advance what I would publish about him. In ordinary circumstances, one cannot publish an identifiable account of a patient without allowing the patient to review the text that will be published and consent to it. But this was not an ordinary circumstance. If he had the right to review the text, neither he nor I could claim it was objective. I saw no way around this ethical problem. I could console myself only with my personal maxim that a person who would avoid all ethical problems must avoid life. I also felt an ethical responsibility to Doctor Snezhnevsky. He had a right to know the result of my examination, whichever way it turned out. I decided to resolve that issue by sharing the findings of my examination with him before I made them public. This decision did not sit well with psychiatric colleagues who participated in the examination of Grigorenko, but it is a practice I have followed in other situations, and I insisted on it here. This, of course, gave Snezhnevsky the opportunity to condemn me and to attempt to undermine the credibility of the report before it was published. As it turned out, he did not use the opportunity in those ways. This is in distinct contrast with my experience with the South African government. An American Psychiatric Association committee which I chaired investigated the treatment of black mental patients in South Africa. When a report of the committee's findings was sent to that government's Department of Health for comments prior to publication, they in effect accused me of being a liar.[42]

These thoughts will suggest something of my "countertransference." But I should also add that although my personal experience was
limited, I had by no means been convinced that all of the Soviet
dissidents who allegedly suffered psychiatric abuse were completely
sane. I was quite open to the possibility that Grigorenko was paranoid. I
believed that the accounts of Amnesty International were somewhat
partisan and sometimes biased. I had the same impression of Block and
Reddaway's book, *Psychiatric Terror*.[43] Indeed, General Grigorenko's
personal experiences with Soviet psychiatry (though not his reports of
what they did to others) suggest a far less damning view than has gained
credence in the West.

Grigorenko's Psychiatrists

Grigorenko's personal experience with psychiatrists, as reported to
me and as described in his memoirs, was complicated, and the different
psychiatrists behaved quite differently. He despised his first psychiatrist, Margarita Felisovna Taltse. He found her stupid, ignorant, and
unaware of history and politics, although not conniving or abusive.
Alexander Pavlovich, who was his psychiatrist at the Leningrad Special
Psychiatric Hospital, was described in a positive way: "I am especially
grateful to Alexander Pavlovich. He never gave me the feeling that he
perceived me as being with a damaged psyche."[44] More importantly,
Grigorenko told me that throughout his years of psychiatric hospitalization he was *never* given neuroleptic drugs by any psychiatrist. This
report is in sharp contrast with claims made by Amnesty International
and other Soviet critics, who suggest that neuroleptics are routinely
administered to dissidents who are not mentally ill.[45] Further, in his
memoirs Grigorenko described a conversation with a psychiatrist named
Doctor Shestakovich. He reported that Shestakovich explained in good
faith that the first Snezhnevsky/Lunts Commission had reached its
conclusion because "we were seeking a solution which was in your own
interests."[46]

Doctor Shestakovich reportedly told Grigorenko that the Commission was trying to save him from a labor camp, which was far worse than
Grigorenko imagined. "I am convinced that in time you will realize that
the way things were done was better for you."[47] Doctor Timofeyev, the
chief psychiatrist of the Academy of Military Medicine, was described
as having been shocked by what happened to Grigorenko and was
reported to have spoken "very effectively as an expert in favor of my
release."[48] Grigorenko also wrote of his gratitude to Doctor Boris

Yefimovich Kagan, who in his view "played the chief role in the decision" that he was sane following his arrest in Tashkent.

At the subsequent Serbsky Institute Commission which reversed this decision, Grigorenko reports that the room was filled with doctors who "were there to learn."[49] I found this description particularly surprising. If the Commission members believed they were calling a sane man insane, why did they open up their examination in this way? Was it to force the entire staff into a posture of solidarity? If they were helping Grigorenko escape a labor camp, snatching him from the K.G.B., would they have felt safe to let all the staff in on it? One cannot rule out the possibility that the Commission members honestly considered Grigorenko an interesting case, a good "grand rounds" patient. Grigorenko was then sixty-two years old, and would spend the next forty months at the Chernyakhovsk Special Psychiatric Hospital in almost constant solitary confinement. Whatever one may think about the good faith of Soviet psychiatrists, there is simply no justification for thus confining Grigorenko: its only purpose was political. Even during his stay there, although Grigorenko describes many abuses of other patients, he was not personally abused. Indeed, he describes how— outraged by the beatings attendants had given a violent patient—he "karate chopped [the attendant] on the throat with the side of my hand. He fell to the floor. After that they didn't touch Borya [the violent patient]."

I find this story shocking only because Grigorenko was not beaten or drugged on the spot. Clearly he was being treated with very special consideration. After his forty months in the special facility, Grigorenko was returned to an ordinary psychiatric hospital in Moscow. There he remained several months until he finally was discharged. It was during this period that a group of Western psychiatrists visited Soviet institutions to investigate political misuse of psychiatry. Two of them were permitted to visit Grigorenko and to interview him. He insisted on his own interpreter. The hospital refused, and no interview took place. He reports that the hospital prepared a false case history—false because "they inserted mention of serious organic injury to my brain."[50] This "forgery" was given to the Western psychiatrists, and a journalist published details of the case in the German magazine Der Stern. Grigorenko pointed to this as a clear example of the duplicity of Soviet psychiatrists.

This story came to light during his examination in Boston, and ironically it played a significant role in my eventual diagnosis of Grigorenko. The "forged" case history reported that Grigorenko had

had a stroke. Doctor Norman Geschwind, Professor of Neurology at Harvard Medical School, in fact discovered when he examined Grigorenko that there was clear evidence that this report was true. He found turbulent blood flow in the right carotid artery with loss of vision in the right eye and signs of weakness and sensory loss on the left side of the body. However, there was no evidence of any other defect in mental status, nor was there evidence of intellectual deterioration. These findings were confirmed by detailed neuropsychological testing done by Doctor Barbara Pendleton Jones.[51]

Based on these observations of Grigorenko's experiences, I reach certain tentative conclusions. On the positive side, no Soviet psychia-trist gave him neuroleptic drugs and no attempt was made to alter his brain or mind. Psychiatrists participated in no physical abuse, or any other unacceptable practice. As he told me, "the walls were my treatment." Some Soviet psychiatrists may have thought they were helping Grigorenko, that they were supplying the least destructive alternative. Whatever the psychiatrists did was done openly. That is, no attempt was made to evaluate Grigorenko secretly. Grigorenko's claim that Soviet psychiatrists prepared a false case history is no longer tenable. It is regrettable that he did not remove or alter this accusation when his memoirs appeared in English in 1982 and when he knew it to be false.

However, on the bad side, it is clear that Soviet psychiatrists discredited Grigorenko's political activities against his wishes and undermined his sense of personal integrity. It is also clear that even if in good faith they believed he was paranoid, they unnecessarily confined him for forty months in a cramped solitary cell in an institution for the criminally insane. I believe this was done to isolate him for political reasons.

Psychiatrists may claim that his confinement in such an institution was by order of a court. But the question then arises, why did Soviet psychiatrists allow him to remain there for forty months? Why did they not return him to an ordinary psychiatric hospital?

In sum, Grigorenko appears to have been unethically and unfairly confined by "overzealous lackeys of the state," or at least by psychia-trists who tolerated political misuse of psychiatry in order to avoid personal risks to themselves and or to Grigorenko. Grigorenko's own judgment about Soviet psychiatrists is much more critical than what has just been described. His judgment is based on his observations of what he saw done to others, and it repeats all of the charges made by other critics of Soviet psychiatry. In retrospect, he condemns most of the psychiatrists who dealt with him personally, but he does not document that condemnation with new facts.

The Diagnosis

I now turn to the more difficult and crucial question. Was Grigorenko paranoid? When Doctor Geschwind informed him of his findings that Grigorenko had had a stroke, and to that extent the "forged" history was correct, General Grigorenko's reaction was very important. He had repeatedly pointed to the "stroke" as proof that the case history was duplicitous, as were the psychiatrists. If he was a typical paranoid with fixed ideas, he could be expected to resist this information, and perhaps even to accuse Doctor Geschwind of complicity or at least to become suspicious. Instead he instantly acknowledged the symptoms and asked what treatment he should have. He explained that when the partial blindness occurred no one had told him it had been caused by a stroke. This sensible nonparanoid reaction was consistent with my entire psychiatric examination and with the detailed psychological examination carried out by Doctor Irene Stiver, Chief of Psychology at McLean Hospital. She found no evidence of paranoid ideation.

My own interview was intentionally confrontational. I challenged his narcissism, his egocentricity, his suspiciousness, and his theories. He was asked, for example: Why did they pick on you? Why should these important people (Khrushchev and Kosygin) be interested in you? They listened to two hours of tapes of you talking? How do you know that Khrushchev was enraged? Why was Khrushchev so angry at you? Why did they let you leave Russia if all that you say is true? Were you betrayed? Do you consider yourself well educated? These questions are taken from the transcript of my examination. He handled all of them with sensible, reasonable, and realistic answers. Not once did I encounter circumstantial responses, ideas of reference, grandiosity, or other paranoid trends. Indeed, I came away from the interview with a genuine feeling of admiration for the General.

The crucial question, of course, was why he gave the fateful speech criticizing Khrushchev, and why did he persist in acts of civil disobedience, destroying his career and knowing, as he claimed, that very little would come of it? I repeat his answer:

> Soviet psychiatrists considered this to be the main evidence for my mental disease, the fact that I entered into this activity knowing of its futility. If American psychiatrists should have the same opinion, I would have to say, I would have to insist, that they are wrong. There

are conditions in which one feels, in which I for example would feel it absolutely impossible to continue in anything like that without [making the speech] otherwise I would consider myself . . . I would lose self respect.

And later he said,

I'm trying to help you, Doctor Stone, to understand me. If it so happens that even in the view of American psychiatrists the readiness to risk one's life is the evidence of mental illness, well then, I'm probably a madman.

I do not believe that any psychiatrist reading the transcript of my interview or the other psychiatric interviews conducted by Doctor Lawrence Kolb and Walter Reich would find evidence of paranoid ideation. A standardized interview following the Spitzer-Endicott Psychiatric Status Schedule, which yields a computerized and weighted scale of psychopathology, was videotaped by Doctor Kolb in New York. None of the reviewers of that interview, including Dr. Jeanne Endicott, diagnosed paranoia. Computerized analysis of the psychiatric status schedule confirmed Dr. Kolb's diagnosis of no mental disorder. After the many examinations of Grigorenko were completed, I felt comfortable to say that in my opinion Grigorenko was not then paranoid and never had been. The summary of the mental status examination was:

General Grigorenko shows no evidence of paranoid personality, paranoid ideation, or paranoid schizophrenia. His sensorium is clear, his judgment is good, his affect is appropriate. He has good insight into his personality and his situation. He relates well, has considerable presence, and is an intelligent and witty man. Although he is deeply committed to his political and moral posture, he has perspective and even a sense of humor about his activities. His facial paralysis and sensorimotor difficulties suggest a cerebral atherosclerotic process.

I sent the complete protocol of my examination to Doctor Snezhnevsky. His response was as follows (the text of the letter is verbatim):

14 March 1979

Prof. Alan A. Stone,
Harvard University,
Langdell Hall,
Harvard Law School,
Cambridge, Mass. 02138.

Dear Dr. Stone:

Thank you for the results of your examination concerning P. Grigorenko that you have sent to us. However due to an absence of a direct contact with the patient, it would inevitably be formalistic. The above mentioned evaluation lacks the description of the patient's personality development, the peculiarities of its reaction to social events. Judging by the medical history of the Serbski Institute during the period preceding P. Grigorenko's reformist activities it was noted that P. Grigorenko being rather active and industrious demonstrated an intensification of an overestimation of his knowledge and abilities, arrogance and lack of control typical for him. In your examination you repeatedly refer to the absense of paranoid signs in the patient and first of all of a schizophrenic genesis. As it follows from the medical history, the staff of Serbski Institute never presumed the existence of this disease in P. Grigorenko. The state was always, qualified as (according to the modern terminology: paranoial personality develop-ment and the traditional one—paranoi originarie). It developed gradu-ally in P. Grigorenko's middle age and manifested itself in reformist activities to restore "the purity of Leninism" and to solve the national question. During the last years of his stay in this country the tension of his activities was reduced to some extent perhaps due to the aging process and atherosclerosis, which is confirmed by the mood lability, euphoria. It is more than difficult to speak of the degree of P. Grigorenko's pathological claims by the essense and ideology of his activities not knowing all the features of the community life in his native land. Kraepelin who described paranoia as a separate nozological unit, wrote: "From the clinical point of view the grouping of pathological picture of a disease is most difficult for there are as many forms of this disease as the patients themselves." Your categorical statement that P. Grigorenko lacks the signs of paranoial pathology, which, as it is known even from the text-books, is detected with a great difficulty (moreover through the interpreter) may only indicate to your enviable courage.

Sincerely yours,

A.V. Snezhnevsky,
Director,
Institute of Psychiatry,
AMS USSR.

The reader should be reminded that Soviet psychiatrists in Tash-kent, "knowing all the features of the community life in his native land," found no "paranoial personality development." This letter also suggests that our examination looked first of all to "a schizophrenic genesis." As the summary mental status indicates, our examination looked for all disorders in which paranoid symptoms are a feature and found none. However, Professor Snezhnevsky is correct that my report did not contain "a description of the patient's personality develop-ment." Such a description was contained in reports prepared by other examiners. It may be appropriate, however, to make some further comments about Grigorenko's personality development from my own psychodynamic perspective.

At the time of my report, Grigorenko's memoirs had not been published in English. The translated version was published in 1982, and I was able to read it before writing this account. Grigorenko was the middle child among three sons, and his mother died when he was three. His father's second wife left the children after a year, when the father was drafted into World War I. Grigorenko had little mothering, important losses, and much emotional deprivation, and in compensation he was much attached to his brothers. He lived a peasant's hard life, and there was much hard labor and little time for play. As he says himself, he had no childhood. But the three brothers were apparently good students and made their way adapting to the changes in their society.

As a child he was quite religious, but in adolescence Grigorenko exchanged religion for communism. His adolescent identity was as a devoted member of the Communist Youth League. Again life was hard, there was much deprivation and famine, and he witnessed a great deal of violence. But he persevered as a believing communist and entered the military. His subsequent career in the military was particularly important to his adult identity. He prided himself on being a professional soldier, a hard worker and an honorable man. He became a master of the science of military strategy. His first marriage was loveless; what was important at that time was that they were both true communists. But despite his early emotional deprivations, he was not incapable of love. He loved his children, and he is deeply devoted to his second wife. He is in every way a self-made man, a survivor who pulled himself up by his own bootstraps.

Like many self-made men, he is also righteous. He made it the hard way and resents those who lied and schemed to get ahead. He has a strong superego, and he is moralistic. He clearly despises politicians who pretend to be war heroes—not just because they are dishonest, but because it is an insult to his own identity. He prides himself on being sensible, disciplined, and hard-working, and he despises stupidity, lack of discipline, freeloading, and corruption. He clearly saw Khrushchev, Kosygin, and Brezhnev as displaying the latter characteristics. I believe that Grigorenko thought that he was a better man than they were. In his mind they were neither heroes of the war nor were they true followers of Lenin. Grigorenko was also a man with a temper. The incident in which he struck the attendant at the Chernyakhovsk Special Psychiatric Hospital was not an isolated event. He describes other instances in his memoirs when he spoke out and hit out in anger, particularly righteous and self-righteous anger. He was also a persistent, perhaps even a stubborn, man. He was able to throw himself into his work when all around him there was conflict, purge, and counterpurge. He could do this even when others had become cynical and concerned only about self interest. His image of himself was as someone who solved problems and not as someone who adapted to the situation. He would pursue his work and his integrity even when it meant struggling against the current. Through most of his military career, work was his only response to the duplicity and corruption he saw around him. His self righteousness was expressed in working even when the work was futile.

I do not believe that this personality sketch of Grigorenko makes him less courageous or more pathological. It is my psychodynamic understanding of his personality after having had the opportunity both to examine him and to read his memoirs. His fateful speech criticizing corruption and Khrushchev was in keeping with his character, as was his subsequent stubborn refusal to recant. He became a dissident in just the way he had been a soldier—determined, hard working, and persistent. He was similarly stubborn and persistent in his efforts to establish his sanity and integrity, whatever the costs. His story is a Russian tragedy because Grigorenko was in fact a decent man and a loyal communist.

THE AMERICAN GENERAL

My discussion of General Walker will of necessity be much briefer. As mentioned, he never consulted me requesting an examination, and he has to my knowledge never published his memoirs. However, there is enough information available to demonstrate the striking parallels and divergences from General Grigorenko's experiences with law and psychiatry.

Major General Edwin Anderson Walker became a well-known figure during the early 1960s. Walker was born in 1909 in Texas, and was raised on a farm there. He attended the U.S. Military Academy at West Point. His military career spanned three decades, and included a series of notable decorations and promotions stemming from his service during World War II and in Korea. Even these bare biographical facts are remarkably similiar to General Grigorenko's history.

In 1959 he took command of the 24th Infantry Division of the United States Army, which was then stationed in Germany. Two years later he launched the "Pro-Blue" indoctrination program[52] that would lead to his official reprimand. One year after that he was ousted from command, following the first among a series of departures from a sterling military career.

Domestically as well, there was a highly visible side to Walker's rise through the military ranks. In 1957 he commanded the Arkansas Military District, and was therefore responsible for the federal troops involved in "Operation Little Rock." Walker openly opposed federal troops' involvement in the desegregation effort, which he termed a "non-military issue."[53] Implicitly, he was criticizing President Eisenhower's decision. Politically, he had long been involved with extreme right-wing political causes and groups. The alleged indoctrination of his troops under the Pro-Blue program was said to involve a significant amount of material similar to that of (if not dispensed by) the John Birch Society.[54]

In 1960, the *Overseas Weekly* publication printed details about General Walker's "indoctrination program." The matter soon came to the attention of the Commander-in-Chief of the Army forces then stationed in Europe. Lieutenant General Frederick J. Brown was assigned Inspector General in the subsequent inquiry. General Brown's panel admonished General Walker for his activities in connection with the Pro-Blue Program. At the same time, Walker's promotion to head the 8th Army Corps was withdrawn.

Desegregation in the Deep South provided the context for one of the most infamous events in Walker's public life: his arrest and subsequent submission to psychiatric evaluation. "Ole Miss," the University of Mississippi, was the site of a spectacular and violent backlash against court-ordered desegregation. Two people died in the resulting furor.[55] Walker, who had already been relieved of his army command, went to Oxford, Mississippi, during the height of the tumult—September 1962. Once there, reported *Life* magazine, Walker "made an extraordinary spectacle of himself, haranguing the mob that assaulted U.S. marshals. . . . The government ordered a psychiatric examination to fathom his bizarre behavior."[56]

Walker was arrested at the scene and charged with assaulting U.S. marshals, resisting arrest, insurrection, and conspiracy.[57] He was also charged with inciting to riot.[58] It was in connection with these charges that the Department of Justice chose to question General Walker's sanity. He had been imprisoned at the Springfield Medical Center for federal prisoners supposedly because only county jails of minimal standards were available for the incarceration of federal prisoners in Mississippi.

Robert Kennedy was then the Attorney General of the United States, and he had been deeply and personally involved in the integration of "Ole Miss," as had been his brother the President of the United States, John F. Kennedy. There can be no doubt that they discussed what to do about General Walker, who had emerged as an important figure in the situation of racial crisis. I would assume, therefore, that when an attorney in the Justice Department called Doctor Charles E. Smith, then Chief Psychiatrist of the Federal Bureau of Prisons, the Attorney General and perhaps the President had agreed on the course of action to be followed.

The attorney asked Doctor Smith "if, on the basis of what he knew of the Walker case, he thought it would be reasonable to make a statement concerning General Walker's condition."[59] We do not know what Doctor Smith knew at that point, but it is clear that he had never personally examined Walker. Doctor Smith, of course, may have already discussed the Walker case by telephone with the staff at the federal facility in Springfield. At any rate, Doctor Smith told the Justice Department that he was prepared to make a statement concerning General Walker's psychiatric condition. That evening the Justice Department delivered to Doctor Smith the following: (1) an Associated Press release describing Walker's activities in Mississippi, (2) a transcript of Walker's testimony about his Pro-Blue indoctrination activities before Congress six months earlier, (3) other news reports about Walker, and (4) Walker's Army medical records.[60]

After studying this material, Doctor Smith prepared an affidavit which sounds remarkably like what Soviet psychiatrists had written about General Grigorenko. "His behavior reflects sensitivity and essentially unpredictable and seemingly bizarre outbursts of the type often observed in individuals suffering with paranoid mental disorder," wrote Smith. Like the Soviet psychiatrists, Doctor Smith suggested that earlier medical complaints and ailments "could be precursors." He concluded that General Walker's behavior "may be indicative of an underlying mental disturbance."[61]

The Justice Department used Doctor Smith's affidavit to request the federal judge to order a psychiatric examination to determine whether Walker was competent to stand trial. Although Walker was already at the Springfield facility, the District Court judge was also asked to designate a suitable hospital where Walker might be committed for this examination. Under American law, the court, the prosecution, and the defense can all request a competency examination. Thus, presumably in Walker's best interest, the Justice Department could impugn his sanity. Section 4244, Title 18, of the United States Code provides that the United States Attorney do this when there is "reasonable cause to believe that a person charged with an offense . . . may be presently insane or otherwise so mentally incompetent as to be unable to understand the proceedings against him or properly to assist in his own defense . . . ."

Presumably, Doctor Smith's affidavit provided the Justice Department with "reasonable cause." They attached it to their motion in support of a competency exam. Such an affidavit is not, however, required under the law. Therefore, it is possible to conclude that the Justice Department wanted to strengthen its hand when impugning Walker's sanity. Judges deciding whether to grant such motions have very little legal guidance. There has been no precise legal definition of the threshold that must be crossed before a competency examination may be ordered. The judge in Walker's case did order the examination, and he ordered that it take place at the Springfield facility where Walker was already confined. This order would probably have meant that Walker's mental condition would have been assessed by government psychiatrists.

Here, however, the American legal system diverges from the Soviet system. Walker's lawyer was able to secure bail the day after the judge's order. Unlike General Grigorenko, who spent years in a special psychiatric facility, General Walker spent one day confined there. This development was not due to the wisdom and objectivity of American psychiatrists, and it was not due to the enlightened provisions of American mental health law. Rather, it was due to the adversarial structure of our legal system, and constitutional safeguards which include the right to a zealous advocate.

With a lawyer to defend him, Walker's rights were protected. The government agreed that Walker would be examined by two psychiatrists, one of them to be selected by the government (but this psychiatrist was not to be a government employee). A government-selected psychiatrist never examined Walker, however. After an examination by Doctor Robert Stubblefield, a psychiatrist apparently selected by General Walker's lawyer, the question of submitting to a government-selected psychiatrist was dropped.

But now Walker's lawyer sought further vindication of his client's sanity. A motion was filed to strike the government's original motion impugning Walker's sanity or, alternatively, to strike Doctor Smith's affidavit. Had the court granted Walker's first request, no psychiatric report, not even the report of Doctor Stubblefield, would have been made to the court. Walker was asking the court to rule that the government had not had reasonable cause to request an examination, or to impugn his sanity. The government opposed these motions and asked for a judicial determination of mental competency.

Doctor Thomas Szasz discussed the Walker case in a book entitled *Psychiatric Justice*, which included a transcript of this proceeding.[62] Walker's lawyers sought to show that the government did not have reasonable cause to request the psychiatric examination.

Two psychiatrists testified for the government at this hearing. Smith testified as to the basis for his affidavit, noting the four separate sources for the recommendations already mentioned: news reports, General Walker's testimony before the Special Preparedness Sub-committee of the Committee on Armed Services,[63] a statement made by a reporter to a Department of Justice official, and Army medical reports on General Walker which noted gastrointestinal problems, headaches and backaches, chronic fatigue and insomnia, and a brief hospitalization in 1960 (a brain tumor was suspected at that time).

The news reports Smith relied on stressed that Walker had "exhorted the public to come to Oxford in large numbers and to join in a coordinated movement, and later it was reported that he led persons against the United States marshals."[64] Similarly, the statement made to the Justice Department officials described Walker as having huddled with a group of students before saying that he stood "ready to fight possibly to the death."[65] Smith's impression was that these reports provided "evidence of behavior out of keeping with that of a person of his station, background, and training."[66]

Smith also termed Walker's beliefs regarding the existence of hidden reasons for his dismissal from his army command to be "sugges-tive of a paranoid trend,"[67] and suggested that Walker harbored "[s]ome abnormal suspicions" with reference to the sources of his ouster.[68] All of this is again startlingly similar to what Soviet psychiatrists said about Grigorenko.

Smith, who was given Walker's Army medical records, apparently had not seen a letter written by a Major General in the army's Medical Corps on September 11, 1961, in which the Major General asserted that, "[o]n the basis of first-hand knowledge, [he] categorically affirm[ed] that medical records of Major General Edwin A. Walker indicate no evidence of brain tumor, central nervous system disease, or any findings of mental disease or mental incompetency."[69]

Manfred Guttmacher, the Dean of American Forensic Psychiatry, was the second witness for the government. He testified that he supported a full psychiatric examination of General Walker. Not surprisingly, Guttmacher based his testimony on many of the same reports and records which Smith claimed to have relied on.

Walker's medical records were apparently quite persuasive for Guttmacher, who, noting the General's bout with encephalitis twelve years earlier, testified that he was "in no position to maintain that [Walker] is now suffering from any residuants from this. On the other hand, it certainly is not conducive to strengthening the nervous system."[70] Guttmacher also stressed Walker's 1960 hospitalization and the clinical observations made immediately prior to the hospitalization, as well as reports of backaches, insomnia, and "prominent nicking of the veins at the arteriovenous junctions."[71]

Guttmacher also echoed Smith's reaction to news accounts which suggested Walker was in Oxford "playing a role that didn't seem to me to show good judgment, and was using tactics and carrying out this mission without the judgment and the control that one would feel appropriate to a man of his type and of his long and very honorable Army record."[72]

Guttmacher read Walker's Senate testimony as providing evidence of mental confusion, feelings of suspicion, and some feelings of grandeur. He cited movie reels of an October press conference as showing slow responses by Walker, and confusion regarding the meaning of questions.[73] He quoted Walker's statement that, "there are thousands going to Mississippi, not only because of my interest" as demonstrating feelings of grandeur.[74]

These feelings of grandeur, Guttmacher testified, were again evident in Walker's Senate testimony when the General stated, "it seems . . . that my case is not merely unusual, but unique. . . . The forces back of it must be extraordinary. These forces cannot be fully identified, but, in general, the Walker case can be recognized as basically a fight between the internationalist left and the nationalist right with control of part of the U.S. Military Establishment at stake."[75] (I might say parenthetically that as a captain in the U.S. Army Medical Corps in 1960, I and all of the other military personnel were required to attend what seemed to me a shockingly right wing indoctrination session that sounded much like General Walker's Senate testimony.)

He also cited Walker's testimony that he had been "framed in a den of iniquity represented by co-existence, no-win, collaborating, soft on communism, national policy," as evidence of confusion and suspicion.[76] Taking all of this evidence together, Guttmacher concluded that there was a "real possibility that there has been a deterioration in the mental processes of General Walker in the past year or two."[77] Thus, Dr. Guttmacher and Dr. Smith resolutely supported the government's claim that there was reasonable cause to impugn the sanity of General Walker, who was charged with crimes arising out of his opposition to the government's policy of racial integration.

The judicial resolution of these matters was artful. The federal judge ruled that the government did have reasonable cause to request the examination. The government was not to be faulted for questioning Walker's sanity. He thereupon accepted Doctor Robert Stubblefield's opinion that Walker was competent to stand trial for the crimes alleged. He added that, "putting aside the psychiatric standpoint," and based on his own opinion as a layman having observed Edwin Walker in the courtroom and on the witness stand, "I would necessarily have found, as I am sure most of you would have, that this man is competent within the meaning of the statute."[78]

It is possible to believe that everyone in the Justice Department and Doctors Smith and Guttmacher acted in good faith. They all believed that General Walker might be mentally ill and that he should be protected against the possibility of being unable to participate in his own defense. But there are other possible explanations for their behavior, including the belief that Doctors Smith and Guttmacher in this instance were "overzealous lackeys of the state." The American Medical Association received "a volume of letters . . . alleging unethical conduct" by Doctor Smith. The story in the *Journal of the American Medical Association* was headlined, "Council answers 2,500 complaints." The council found Smith guilty of no ethical violation. But it did, in light of the incident, warn doctors about being "used as a tool for political purposes."[79] Not unlike Dr. Snezhnevsky's comments, the council of the American Medical Association put the onus for what had happened on the courts. "It is then the Courts' responsibility to evaluate such opinions."[80]

The case of General Walker was filled with political irony. Having been found competent to stand trial, the government was unable to get a Mississippi jury to indict him, and so the case against him was dismissed on January 21, 1963.

The matter was not, however, at a close—least of all in the legal realm. Walker filed several libel suits against major news services, including a two million dollar suit against the Associated Press for its coverage of his part in the Oxford events. Szasz noted that, ironically, an $800,000 judgment against the Associated Press stemmed from the very news report that Doctor Smith listed first in detailing the sources upon which he based his affidavit.[81] General Walker, because he was by legal definition a public figure, lost his judgment on appeal.

Since his 1962 arrest, Walker's name has been linked to a variety of sometimes bizarre events and incidents. In April 1963 he was fired at by a rifleman. Later events made it appear that Presidential assassin Lee Harvey Oswald had been the gunman.[82] In 1965, Walker made news when the Internal Revenue Service claimed he owed nearly four thousand dollars in federal income taxes for 1961.[83] Some would say that this is further proof that he was still being persecuted by the federal government.

In 1969 his right-wing political views again gained a public forum, as he joined forces with John Birch Society leader David Smoot to organize a Texas chapter in support of George Wallace's Presidential candidacy.[84] (Walker had political aspirations of his own, having once filed and lost a bid for the Texas Democratic nomination for Governor.)

In later years he achieved public notice under considerably more ignominious circumstances—circumstances which would lead many psychoanalytically oriented psychiatrists to give credence to Doctors Smith and Guttmacher's diagnoses fifteen years earlier. Walker was arrested twice in Dallas, in 1976 and in 1977, on charges of public lewdness in connection with approaches made to plainclothes police officers in a park restroom.[85]

COMMENTS ON POLITICS AND PARANOIA

Paranoia is one of the most troubling concepts in the psychiatric lexicon. Every psychiatrist with clinical experience knows that the phenomenon is real. Yet every psychiatrist knows or has heard of at least one case in which a person diagnosed as paranoid, with a supposedly false belief system, was in fact telling a true story. Because psychiatrists are not omniscient and because unverifiable beliefs are part of culture and religion, there is always an element of doubt.

There are helpful clinical rules of thumb in distinguishing paranoia from reality. Paranoia may be indicated where the fixed ideas place the ordinary person at the center of a great deal of extraordinary activity by important people; where sexual themes are prominent, where unrelated events are crudely woven into the central idea, where the person's commitment to the ideas is more urgent than anything else in his or her life; where there is obvious projection of personal concerns with seemingly bizarre features, when contradictory evidence has no weight or significance.

But all of these useful clinical indications may be unavailing when, as in this "tale of two generals," the persons involved are important figures and appropriately consider themselves important, when high governmental authorities do involve themselves in those important people's lives, and when apparently unrelated events are related. One also cannot escape the fact that the psychiatrist's judgment about the falseness of a belief system is necessarily related to his own belief system. The psychiatrist does not exist separate from culture.

There are ways, however, to compensate for this culture-bound aspect of our diagnostic judgment. One useful rule of thumb is to ask oneself whether the fixed idea is idiosyncratic to the supposed patient, or if it is shared by others. General Grigorenko's and General Walker's beliefs were not idiosyncratic. Grigorenko's views are shared by many Soviet dissidents, and Walker's views were the opinions of the John Birch Society.

Snezhnevsky and Lunts could have seen that Grigorenko's ideas were not idiosyncratic, but that, of course, would have placed them in the awkward position of giving a certain legitimacy to those views. The same problem confronted Smith and Guttmacher. They would have been saying that racism was the accepted belief of a sane general shared by many sane Americans. It should be emphasized that both generals' "fixed ideas" attacked the most delicate political question of their nation: the corruption of the Soviet Revolution and the racism of the world's greatest democracy. When an important general announces his dissidence or his racism, political wheels start spinning. Surely there were temptations for these psychiatrists to become "overzealous lackeys" or "tool[s] for political purposes," whether to gain favor with the Politburo or with the Kennedy administration.

Against this temptation, these psychiatrists had very little to guide them. As General Grigorenko pointed out himself, the psychiatrists were influenced by the fact that he risked everything to proclaim and propagate his views. Soviet psychiatrists, for example, might privately think that many Soviet citizens believe their government is corrupt and has corrupted the revolution but that sane people are sensible enough to remain silent. Similarly, many American generals may be racists but they are sensible enough not to announce these ideas.

In this perspective it is not the beliefs which are mad; rather, the madness is to announce these ideas in public and to act on them. Thus, to act against self interest because of deep conviction would seem to be a sign of paranoia. Psychiatrists must acknowledge that such is typically our view. Freud noted that there is a continuum of paranoia: people who have paranoid dreams, paranoid fantasies which are easily dismissed, paranoid ideas which cannot be put out of consciousness despite a conscious struggle, and then paranoid ideas as a consuming preoccupation. The gradations are familiar to anyone who has attempted to treat a paranoid patient. Yet such gradations are apparent in any believer. One could as easily describe Christians and Marxists along just such a continuum. The true believer is so much like the false believer—even down to the gleam in the eye.

These questions have tortured psychiatry in this century and the questions are inescapable. But if there are no ready solutions, there are at least sensible compromises. First, a line can be drawn between idiosyncratic fixed ideas and fixed ideas shared with others. Perhaps the term idiosyncratic paranoia should be specifically distinguished from paranoia. Second, a distinction should be made between the forms of idiosyncratic paranoia in which the self is the center of the drama and those forms in which others are also protagonists and victims ("they are poisoning me" versus "they are poisoning us"). Third and last, a distinction should be made between idiosyncratic paranoia with and without bizarre content ("there is a conspiracy against me" versus "there is a conspiracy to use my brain to broadcast sexual ideas").

These distinctions might bring some bright lines to an otherwise ambiguous diagnostic category. When combined with a careful history of the origins of the "paranoia," there will be more solid grounds for the diagnosis. In political cases where there is danger of being an "overzealous lackey" one might draw the line at idiosyncratic paranoia with bizarre content. Such cases would, of course, be closer to schizophrenia. Neither General Grigorenko nor General Walker could have been diagnosed as having idiosyncratic paranoia with bizarre content.

But even if the diagnosis of paranoia were more carefully drawn, there is the question of what legal significance it should be given. My own conclusion is that only idiosyncratic paranoia with bizarre content should count as a mental illness for any legal purpose. This is in the way of a "convention," but it has the virtue that it would draw a brighter line than now exists between mental illness and political dissent. It is based on the assumption that idiosyncratic fixed ideas with bizarre content are least likely to be political beliefs. And it is based on the premise that an essential characteristic of madness is that the person is isolated in his belief system.

This convention runs counter to the Soviet diagnostic scheme and to the nosological theories of most Western psychiatrists. It also runs counter to current legal theories which would exclude all diagnostic criteria from legal considerations. Its virtue is that it recognizes that madness is a social construct, and that recognition operates as a constraint in establishing the convention of legally significant madness. The convention is not perfect. It may not even be workable. However, it puts the right questions on the agenda for discussions of political misuse of psychiatry and the diagnosis of paranoia.

CONCLUDING REMARKS

The cases of General Grigorenko and General Walker lead one to the conclusion that the difference in their fates has less to do with psychiatry than it has to do with law. Psychiatrists in America chafe under the increasing intrusions of lawyers and judges. Many of them believe that adversarial testimony is a bad thing and would opt for a Soviet-style commission. They resent the time spent in court, the many legal appeals, and the safeguards which include the right to a jury trial. All of this seems unnecessary until we look at the question of political misuse of psychiatry. It is the American legal system's constitutional safeguards which protected General Walker. It is the absence of such safeguards that led to the "psychiatric terrorism" in General Grigorenko's case.

The American system of law was designed to protect the citizen's rights against the state. The Soviet system of government was designed to reconstruct the social order. The American legal system is adversarial. The citizen's lawyer is a zealous advocate against the state. The Soviet legal system puts the welfare of the people's revolution ahead of the person. In the end, these fundamental differences influence everything, even the political misuse of psychiatry.

We can honestly criticize the Soviet psychiatrists who confined Grigorenko in a special hospital for the criminally insane. But the rest of their actions seem less reprehensible, and their motives less clear, when one has a better appreciation of their legal system and the realities of their situation. At worst, they have been overzealous lackeys of the state. At best, they really believed that they were acting in General Grigorenko's best interests. There is evidence for both conclusions. The same can be said for Doctor Smith and Doctor Guttmacher.

Finally, a word about the similarities is in order. Although Soviet and American laws are very different, they both permit the govern-ment's lawyers to raise the question of a criminal defendant's sanity. This gives the government's lawyers in both countries an opportunity to impugn the sanity of the defendant. This is a powerful weapon against political dissidents. The stigma of insanity is real in the political context. In the Soviet Union, many citizens to this day may think of Grigorenko as the crazy general just as many American citizens remember General Walker only as that crazy general. In both countries, the reasons for the laws which permit lawyers for the government to question a defendant's sanity are benevolent, and benevolence is the practical result in most cases. However, at least in America, where every alleged criminal is entitled to a lawyer, one might well ask, why not let the defendant and his lawyer decide that question? At the very least, the ethical guidelines for prosecutors should caution against raising the issue of madness in political cases, and psychiatrists should bend over backwards to avoid complicity and the danger of becoming overzealous lackeys.

REFERENCES

1. Wing, Psychiatry in the Soviet Union, *British Medical Journal*, March 9, 1974, p. 433.

2. Working Group on the Internment of Dissenters in Mental Hospitals, *Dr. Semyon Gluzman: The Imprisoned Conscience of Soviet Psychiatry* (London, England, 1977).

3. *See, e.g.*, Amnesty International, *Political Abuse of Psychiatry in the U.S.S.R., An Amnesty International Briefing* (1983) and Amnesty International, *Prisoners of Conscience in the U.S.S.R., Their Treatment and Conditions* (1975).

4. Criminal Code of the Russian Soviet Federal Socialist Republic, Translated by H. J. Berman and J. W. Spindler, in *Soviet Criminal Law and Procedure* (Harvard University Press, 1972).

5. *Lancet*, April 11, 1981, p. 820.

6. *See* International Association on the Political Use of Psychiatry, *Soviet Political Psychiatry, The Story of the Opposition* (London, 1983).

7. *See* Pivnicki, Ethics and Psychiatry, *Canadian Psychiatric Association Journal*, Vol. 23, p. 337 (1978).

8. Wing, *op. cit.*

9. Anonymous, *The Soviet State and Psychiatry, A Chronicle of Human Rights in the U.S.S.R.* (Khronika Press, No. 30, April–June 1978).

10. Both Lunts and Morozov supposedly have connections with the K.G.B.

11. Amnesty International Secretariat, *External Press Release*, August 1, 1977.

12. International Association on the Political Use of Psychiatry, *Information Bulletin* No. 7 (1983).

13. *Ibid.*

14. *See, e.g.*, Bazelon, Introduction, G. V. Morozov and La M. Kalashnik, *Forensic Psychiatry* (approved translation) (International Arts and Sciences Press: 1970). *See also*, Babayan, Legal Aspects of Psychiatry in the Soviet Union, *Psychiatric Annals*, Vol. 8, pp. 37–50 (1978).

15. W. A. Veenhoven, ed., *Case Studies on Human Rights and Fundamental Freedoms, A World Survey*, Vol. II (Kluwer Academic, 1975) pp. 538–547.

16. Heston, "The Genetics of Schizophrenic and Schizoid Disease," *Science*, January 16, 1970, p. 249.

17. Ghadirian, Some Recent Advances in the Study and Treatment of Schizophrenia in the Soviet Union, *The Psychiatric Journal of the University of Ottawa*, Vol. 2, pp. 112–116 (1977).

18. Wing, *op. cit.*

19. *Ibid.*

20. *See* International Association on the Political Use of Psychiatry, *Information Bulletin* No. 6 (1983).

21. *See* H. Fireside, *Political Abuse of Psychiatry in the U.S.S.R.*, Paper delivered at Annual Meeting of the American Political Science Association (1978).

22. P. G. Grigorenko, *The Grigorenko Papers*, translation (Westview Press, 1976).

23. *Ibid.*

24. The General assumed his Ukranian name, Petro, in place of the Russian name Pyotr, when his Soviet citizenship was revoked.

25. P. G. Grigorenko, *Memoirs* (W. W. Norton and Co., 1982), p. 242.

26. *Ibid.*, p. 253.

27. *Ibid.*, p. 251.

28. *Ibid.*, p. 263.

29. *Ibid.*, p. 272.

30. *Ibid.*, p. 278.

31. *Ibid.*, p. 286.

32. *Ibid.*, p. 288.

33. *Ibid.*, p. 288.

34. *Ibid.*, p. 290.

35. Such diagnoses ordinarily are annulled only upon the hospital's application. *Ibid.*, p. 303.

36. Grigorenko, *Memoirs, op. cit.*, p. 347.

37. Transcript of Stone examination, p. 1.

38. Grigorenko, *Memoirs, op. cit.*, p. 395.

39. *See generally*, A. A. Stone, *Mental Health and Law: A System in Transition*, Chapter 12, (National Institute of Mental Health, 1975).

40. Grigorenko, *Memoirs, op. cit.*, p. 428.

41. *Ibid.*, p. 449–450.

42. Department of Health, South Africa, *Comments on the Report of the Committee to visit South Africa: The American Psychiatric Association* (1979).

43. S. Block and P. Reddaway, *Psychiatric Terror: How Soviet Psychiatry is used to Suppress Dissent* (Basic Books, 1977).

44. Grigorenko, *Memoirs, op. cit.*, p. 300.

45. *See, e.g.*, Report of the International Association on the Political Use of Psychiatry, *Soviet Political Psychiatry* (1983). *See also* Soviet Abuse of Political Prisoners,

Hearings before the Subcommittee on International Organizations, 94th Congress, 2d Sess. 11 (1976) (L. Plyushch, Testimony on Psychiatric Abuse of Political Prisoners).

46. Grigorenko, *Memoirs, op. cit.*, p. 299.

47. *Ibid.*, p. 300.

48. *Ibid.*, p. 303.

49. *Ibid.*, p. 399.

50. *Ibid.*, p. 426.

51. Tests administered: WAIS (Partial), Bender Gestalt, Benton Visual Retention, Raven Colored Progressive Matrices, Rey Auditory Verbal Learning, Wisconsin, card sorting, controlled word association, logical memory and visual reproduction subtests from Wechsler Memory Scale I, Neuropsychological screen examinations (portions).

52. The Pro-Blue Education and Training Program (so-named to be synonymous with "Anti-Red," a term used in battle training exercises) stressed to Walker's troops the importance of education about the purported evils of "overt and covert Communist methodology," and included a detailed exposition of the importance of morale, religion, and discipline. *See* program outline, in I. McAnally, The Decision of General Walker, *Walker, Censorship and Survival* (The Bookmailer, 1961), pp. 29–52.

53. Text of statement to U.S. Senate Armed Services Committee, reprinted, *ibid.*, at p. 21.

54. McAnally claims that the material distributed was later acknowledged by the Secretary of the Army as not having any connection to the John Birch Society, McAnally, *op. cit.*, p. 60.

55. *See* R. Kluger, *Simple Justice* (Vintage Books, 1975), p. 755.

56. *Life*, October 12, 1962, p. 42.

57. *New York Times*, September 30, 1962.

58. P. A. Carmichael, *The South and Segregation* (Public Affairs Press, 1965), p. 15.

59. Judicial Council of the American Medical Association, General Walker and Doctor Smith, *Journal of the American Medical Association*, July 6, 1963, pp. 36–37.

60. *Ibid.*

61. *Ibid.*

62. T. Szasz, *Psychiatric Justice* (Macmillan, 1979).

63. *Military Cold War Education and Speech Review Policies, Hearings before the Senate Committee on Armed Services, Subcommittee on Special Preparedness* (Part 4), 87th Cong., 2d Sess. 1839 (1962).

64. Transcript of Direct Examination and Cross Examination of psychiatric witnesses, reproduced in Szasz, *op. cit.*, p. 191.

65. *Ibid.*, p. 191.

66. Judicial Council of the American Medical Association, *op. cit.*, p. 37.

67. Transcript, in Szasz, *op. cit.*, p. 198.

68. *Ibid.*, p. 197.

69. *Ibid.*, p. 195.

70. *Ibid.*, p. 200.

71. *Ibid.*, p. 201.

72. *Ibid.*, p. 203.

73. *Ibid.*, pp. 202–203.

74. *Ibid.*, p. 203.

75. *Ibid.*, p. 211–212.

76. *Ibid.*, pp. 202.

77. *Ibid.*, p. 203.

78. Judicial Council of the American Medical Association, *op. cit.*, p. 37.

79. *Ibid.*

80. *Ibid.*

81. Szasz, *op. cit.*, p. 221.

82. *See New York Times*, April 12, 1963. *See also New York Times*, December 7, 1963, and October 13, 1977. (Oswald's widow proclaimed her feelings of guilt for not having informed police that her husband had fired at Walker.)

83. *New York Times*, October 21, 1965.

84. *New York Times*, March 17, 1969.

85. *New York Times*, July 9, 1976; August 17, 1976; and March 18, 1977.

II

Psychiatry and Violence

THIS CHAPTER IS DIVIDED into three brief sections. In the first, I describe and criticize how the Criminal Justice System in the United States deals with violence and crime. In the second part, I describe and criticize how psychiatry attempted to help the law deal with violence and crime. In the third brief and final section, I suggest two lessons for the future relationship between law and psychiatry in dealing with violence.

The United States is obsessed with violence and crime. In New York City, which I shall use as an example, estimates are that one out of every three people over age 15 has an illegal handgun. The FBI reports that New Yorkers own two million illegal handguns. The United States manufactures two million handguns a year, and we import hundreds of thousands from foreign suppliers.[1] Unable to disarm ourselves at home, is there any wonder that we are unable to agree to international disarmament? Handguns, of course, contribute only a small part to our crime and our violence. Our inner cities have periodically erupted in racial rioting, looting, burning, and destruction.[2] There are parts of New York and other major cities which still look like a war zone. Violence within our families seems to be increasing requiring the creation of a new Presidential Commission, and there is, of course, mayhem on our highways with fifty thousand people being killed each year.[3]

Some years ago Karl Menninger, commenting on this epidemic of crime and violence, reminded us that "violence is as American as apple pie." Menninger's view might be thought of as an ironic comment on human nature, or at least human nature in the United States. Sigmund Freud is reported to have remarked to Ernest Jones that the United States is gigantic, but a gigantic mistake.[4] Whatever the peculiar failings of the United States may be, it is clear that Freud and Menninger share the view that there is a potentially violent side to human nature, the beast in man which must be tamed by culture and civilization. When culture and civilization fail, the innate violence comes out. This is Freud's explicit vision in *Civilization and Its Discontents*,[5] and it is implicit in his structural theory of the ego, the id, and the superego. I shall have more to say about this bleak vision, but I want briefly to contrast it with another vision of violence.

At about the same time Karl Menninger was reminding us that violence was as American as apple pie, two neurosurgeons and a psychiatrist at Harvard Medical School were offering a different theory. After the inner city riots of the 1960s, they wrote to the *New York Times* and the *Journal of the American Medical Association* suggesting that despite the recent looting, rioting, and burning in our inner cities there had, in fact, been relatively little actual violence as measured by killings and serious injuries. They speculated that perhaps some or most of the actual violence had been caused by persons suffering from brain abnormalities particularly disorders of the limbic system.[6] Some readers of these letters took them as ignoring the political and revolutionary significance of these violent events. Remember that in a political discourse, the difference between a revolutionary and a terrorist can be a matter of personal ideology. The Harvard Medical School letters suggested that—be they revolutionaries, terrorists, or policemen—if violent, they were possibly brain damaged. This brought down on the Harvard physicians charges of racism and started a controversy that has not yet been forgotten. Two of these doctors, Mark and Ervine, published a monograph called *Violence and the Brain*.[7] They argued that Freud's bleak vision of human nature, shared by Konrad Lorenz, was wrong, as were all other theorists who posited an instinctual aggressive or violent drive. There was not a human instinct for violence. The only instinct, in their more optimistic view, was the classic evolutionary fight or flight instinct for survival, which is set off when, and only when, any animal is confronted with danger.[8] Diseases of the limbic system could distort the fight/flight instinct and set off the trigger of violence in the amygdala of the brain. They described as a possible cure for violence stereotaxic surgery of the amygdala in patients with temporal lobe conditions. Their countervision to theories of instinctual violence is that violence, or at least *much* violence, is a disease of the brain and not basic to the innate human condition. One could mention other theories of violence: for example, that violence is like all other behaviors—learned by social reinforcement. For now, however, I would like the reader to keep in mind just two caricatured positions: that violence is innate in and proceeds from human nature and the counterthesis that violence is a disease of the brain.

THE LAW AND ITS FAILINGS

With this dichotomy to orient our thinking, let us look at some empirical facts about violence in the United States and the role of law and its failings. In the United States, violent crime has increased substantially over the past three decades.[9] Wolfgang, a criminologist, has studied two cohorts of young men in Philadelphia: one cohort consisted of boys who were all born in 1945; the other, boys who were all born in 1958. He compared the rate of crime in the two cohorts. The younger cohort, growing up in the 1960s and 1970s, committed three times as many killings, twice as many rapes, six times as many robberies, and twice as many aggravated assaults.[10] Some criminologists have suggested that crime and violence will eventually go down in the United States, but only because the birthrate is dropping and eventually the population of males between the ages of 15 and 25 (considered the most prone to violent crimes) will decrease in absolute numbers.[11]

Now, how has the United States' legal system dealt with all this violence and crime? The majority of crimes, of course, result in no arrest. Although there is variation depending on the kind of crime, the generalization holds. The police rarely solve crimes in the manner that readers of detective stories might think. They depend on informants and people giving themselves up.[12] Nonetheless, the best estimates by Greenwood[13] are that in recent years, the police have made about one and one half million felony arrests annually. Felonies are the more serious crimes as contrasted with misdemeanors, but of course they are not all violent crimes. Are these one and one half million arrestees guilty? According to criminal defense lawyers, a realistic guess is that the vast majority of them are in fact guilty of some felony, if not exactly the one

with which they are charged. Hollywood, television, and the media like
to emphasize the frequency with which police arrest totally innocent
people. But these are uncommon exceptions according to knowledgeable
observers. Most criminal defense lawyers will devote their professional
careers to defending guilty people. What happens to the million and a
half arrestees who, though guilty in fact, are by law presumed to be
innocent? A third of these arrestees have their charges dropped. Of the
million who remain, only 50 percent are convicted, and of that 50
percent (or 500,000 felons), only about 80,000 go to prison.[14]

   Why is it that across the United States only five percent of arrested
felons go to prisons? There are many reasons; some of them are sensible
reasons, others are not. Recently, a group of prosecutors had been
working with the Harvard Criminal Justice Center. Prosecutors from
the federal, state, and local governments were represented. The general
consensus of these prosecutors is that they lack adequate financial and
legal resources to prosecute all of the criminals who are arrested.[15]
Increasingly, in the United States, our police feel trapped between the
criminals on one side, whose violence they cannot control, and the
prosecutors on the other side, who are unable to prosecute many of the
criminals the police do manage to arrest. The emerging prosecutorial
strategy is to get the maximum bang for the buck.[16] One way to do this is
by selecting for special prosecutorial attention those felony defendants
who supposedly have committed a disproportionate number of violent
offenses.

   A word should be said about these multiple violent offenders who
are targeted for special prosecutorial attention. Recent studies by the
Rand Corporation, using self reports (interviews and questionnaire
surveys of prisoners in California, Michigan, and Texas) suggest that a
small percentage of the prisoners have committed a disproportionate
amount of the serious crimes.[17] The Rand studies are corroborated by
Wolfgang's cohort studies. There seems to be a small subgroup of
"violent predators," perhaps less than 10 percent of convicted criminals, who commit as many as 40 percent of the crimes.[18] These "violent
predators" are the target of special prosecutorial attention. However, to
identify the violent predator is not always easy, and it requires doing a
number of things which are objectionable to civil libertarians. For
example, violent predators begin their criminal careers as juveniles.
Documenting their predatory violence so that they can be prosecuted
before their career has taken its toll of victims might require that
prosecutors have access to juvenile records. Civil libertarians in the
United States do not take kindly to this. They would prefer that juvenile

records be sealed and that the person be given a fresh start as an adult at age 18. Furthermore, since many criminal predators travel from state to state, identifying them requires computerized information that is accessible from state to state, including juvenile records. Lastly, there is the question whether the many arrests that do not end in conviction should be computerized and used in this way, given the law's presumption of innocence.[19]

There are certain other ways to identify those who may make a career as violent predators, but these are based on characteristics having to do with status rather than criminal acts and are therefore equally troubling to civil libertarians. They include such things as being young, unemployed, and a substance abuser. Psychiatrists will recognize that criteria identifying the violent predator are similar to criteria of sociopathic personality disorder in the *Diagnostic and Statistical Manual of Mental Disorders* (Third Edition) (DSM-III). Of particular interest is the fact that our criteria also emphasize onset before age 15. However violent predators are legitimately identified, the current progressive prosecution strategy in the United States is to maximize the bang for the buck by trying to "incapacitate" them. Critics say there is little new in this, since prosecutors have always gone after "bad guys" anyway, and they cite studies which suggest that such prosecutorial strategy produces no bigger bang for the buck. Furthermore, establishing special prosecutorial units with more resources to go after the violent predators may destroy the morale of the other prosecutors.[20]

Beyond civil libertarian and professional bureaucratic objections, I have my own personal reservations about the pragmatic value of this approach. There is good reason to believe that many street criminals are aware of how prosecutors work. When the word goes out on the street that the District Attorney only goes after the people who commit X number of armed robberies, there will then be an inducement to rational criminals to commit up to $X - 1$ crimes. And if a substantial number do commit up to $X - 1$ crimes, selective incapacitation could result in an overall increase in violence. With or without new prosecutorial strategies, the legal system I have been describing to you is, I think, a failure. It fails to protect the public if each year 1,420,000 felony arrestees are released back onto the streets. Again, consider New York City. Although the national average is 5 percent, 99 percent of felony arrests in New York City do not result in the arrestee's actually serving a sentence in a state prison.[21] Who are the arrested felons who go back on the streets? One group consists of men convicted for the first time of armed robbery. These are men who have put a gun to someone's head, preferably a tourist, and uttered some equivalent of the famous line, "Your money or your life." The knowledgeable armed robber likes to pick tourists because it is unlikely that a tourist will be willing to return to the city to testify against him. Thus, in the unlikely event that he is caught and arrested, the charges will be dropped for lack of evidence. Now take the unlikely case in which the armed robber is caught and is convicted in New York City. Such first conviction armed robbers are routinely given suspended sentences—they are back on the streets.[22] I have no doubt that many of those who are *legally* defined as first offenders are actually multiple offenders and this is simply the first time they have been caught.

I want to describe another New York statistic to you. The Harvard Criminal Justice Center, in a report based on the work of the Vera Institute of Justice, found that in one year in New York City there were 95,000 good felony arrests for violent crimes, rape, murder, armed robbery, etcetera. Of these 95,000 arrests, only one half of one percent resulted in an actual criminal trial.[23] You have already heard how limited prosecutorial resources are. Even if those resources were increased a hundred times, it would not be nearly enough if every arrested criminal demanded his constitutional right to a trial before a jury of his peers. The American Criminal Justice System is ready to collapse under its own weight. The criminals, if they ever organized themselves into a union and refused to plea bargain, could bring the whole enterprise to its knees. My colleague, Alan Dershowitz, has described the courthouse as resembling a Turkish bazaar more than a hall of justice.[24] And no wonder—prosecutors as well as defense lawyers are scrambling to make bargains; they have no choice.

I said that the Criminal Justice System fails to protect the public, but all this deal-cutting results in another kind of failure, a corruption of the public's sense of justice. Not only are the victims of violent crimes appalled by these deals that send criminals who have terrorized them back to the streets; the 80,000 criminals who do go to prison also end up feeling that they got a bad deal. Many of them can tell you about someone who committed far worse crimes than they did who beat the rap or whose lawyer got them a better deal, or who had more money to pay for high powered lawyers. Furthermore, given the limited prosecutorial resources, it is easy for convicted criminals, even hardened Mafia types, to feel that the District Attorney was out to get them rather than to acknowledge their guilt and the justice of their convic-tion. This psychology is widespread. Remember Richard Nixon's re-sponse to the Watergate prosecutions for a "third rate burglary." Imagine how the Reverend Sun Myung Moon must feel about the motives of the prosecutors charging him with being a tax criminal. In one sense these defendants are correct. For example, given all of the felons arrested and all of the terrible things they have done, to spend millions of dollars prosecuting Reverend Moon is the setting of a priority to get him and not to get others (perhaps to get him because of his religious proselytizing and not just because he is believed to be a tax criminal). Thus, our Criminal Justice System fails to protect the public, and the system itself corrupts the very notion of even-handed justice. I have not yet even discussed its greatest failings.

It is time for some more statistics. The Justice Department has recently reported that there are now 1,300,000 United States citizens who have been convicted of a crime and are currently on probation. Almost a quarter of a million Americans have served time in prison and are now out on parole,[25] and over 400,000 people are confined in prisons.[26] The total is over two million. Think about it—in the United States of America, even with all of the difficulty it takes to get arrested and to get convicted, one out of every one hundred Americans is a convicted criminal. Just to state the numbers, two million—one in a hundred, is to recognize that the Criminal Justice System cannot rehabilitate, cannot protect, cannot deter, cannot supervise—in short, cannot achieve any of the supposed goals of criminal punishment. No wonder that the scientists at Rand Corporation, based on their studies, now urge prosecutorial strategies in which the primary goal is the incapacitation of violent predators.

Let us now consider briefly the situation of the over 400,000 Americans who are incapacitated. It will come as no surprise that blacks and Hispanics are vastly overrepresented. And even though it is factually correct that these minorities commit a disproportionate percentage of violent crimes, there is still convincing evidence that when their sentences are compared with those of equally violent whites, there seems to have been bias and racism in the sentencing.[27] It should also not surprise you that our prisons are filled with racial violence and that there are race riots in prisons, both among prisoners and between prisoners and guards. Prisoners kill, maim, and rape each other.[28] Our prisons are vastly overcrowded. In the state of Massachusetts some facilities now hold three times as many prisoners as their original maximum capacities. Several prisoners who have escaped from prison, been recaptured, and then been tried for the offense of escaping have defended themselves on a theory of self defense, necessity, or duress—they were forced to escape to avoid being raped, beaten, or killed.[29] Lawyers who have studied these cases claim that if similar undisputed facts were offered as a defense in any context other than a prison escape, the defendants would be found not guilty. Courts simply will not acknowledge the horrible reality that exists in many of our prisons. But that horrible reality has been acknowledged by a few Federal judges who in certain instances have found conditions bad enough to constitute cruel and unusual punishment. Some of these judges, in order to deal with overcrowding, have required states to release prisoners early.[30]

The evidence is overwhelming. It seems patently obvious that our prisons are a failure, and it is clear that the overcrowding has affected the whole system of justice. Convicted criminals must be given proba-tion because there is no room in the prison. And the ultimate irony of the Criminal Justice System is that, for those who do go to prison, the real punishment is inflicted not by the state, but by the other prisoners who will rape, kill, and torment them. Such a legal system mocks the no-tion of justice and undermines any sense that a criminal might have of being morally responsible for a violent crime.

I would describe the system of criminal justice in the United States as triage justice. The judge is like a doctor dealing with a disaster where victims overwhelm the available resources. So triage justice means using the limited resources to confine the worst offenders or selecting political targets that help prosecutors get reelected. Triage justice is, of course, most apt to be practiced in our major cities, where most of the crime takes place. For example, in New York State there were 2,128 murders in 1981, 1,826 of which occurred in New York City—five murders a day requires triage justice.[31] Ironically, for any theory of deterrence, this means that felons arrested in high-crime areas are less likely to go to prison than those in low-crime areas.

After this account you can understand my response to recent complaints in the United States that psychiatry and the insanity defense were corrupting the system of justice. My response was that the insanity defense is a pimple on the nose of justice but the patient is dying of congestive heart failure. You may also understand why I have criticized the attempts of legal activists in the United States who want to reform the mental health system by making it over in the image of the Criminal Justice System.[32]

PSYCHIATRY'S ATTEMPTS TO HELP THE LAW

But it is now time to look at the attempts of psychiatry to guide the Criminal Justice System in its efforts to deal with violent crime. During the twentieth century, a number of psychiatrists have suggested important legal reforms of the Criminal Justice System. All of these reforms were based on the assumption that many violent criminals are sick and that they should be diagnosed and treated rather than punished. At the very least, psychiatrists argued, these sick criminals should be confined in secure therapeutic facilities rather than prisons. All of these reforms exaggerated either psychiatry's ability to cure violence or its prospects of finding a cure for violence. Manfred Guttmacher is, perhaps, the most notable example. Under his leadership the state of Maryland enacted statutes which created a new kind of legal confinement for the so-called defective delinquents.[33] Earlier statutes in other states had focused only on the sexual psychopath. Guttmacher's idea was to expand the category to include all violent mentally ill criminals who, under the "Defective Delinquent" statutes he advocated, were to be given day-to-life sentences—confined until cured. The result of the Maryland defective delinquent statute, like other similar statutes, was to foster a third kind of institution. On the one hand there were prisons, on the other hand there were mental hospitals. In between there were institutions for the criminally insane, which now also would be used for sexual psychopaths and for defective delinquents. These in-between institutions provided what I have described as quasi-criminal confinement. These institutions, of course, are the American equivalents of the special psychiatric facilities in the Soviet Union as described in the first chapter.

Psychiatry in the United States is typically seen as harassed by constitutional litigation and regulation—I have often so described it. But it was because of these quasi-criminal institutions and the abuses that occurred in them that legal precedents were set and, based on those precedents, the legal attack on psychiatry in the United States began. Before describing these legal developments, let me point out that quasi-criminal institutions by most accounts have been a terrible failure, not only in the sense that they often failed to offer meaningful treatment, but also because they typically created an environment worse than prisons or mental institutions.[34]

Under quasi-criminal confinement, involving day-to-life sentences, treatment became a con game in which patients pretended to be cured in order to be freed. In short, the attempt to treat violent offenders in special institutions failed as treatment and failed as justice.

Let me turn briefly to how the legal attack on psychiatry began in those institutions. Psychiatry, of course, had welcomed, indeed helped, to create Judge David Bazelon's expanded insanity defense in the famous Durham decision. As a result, many defendants in the District of

Columbia who would have gone to prison or on probation were found not guilty by reason of insanity and went instead to the John Howard Pavilion of St. Elizabeth's Hospital, where John Hinckley, the would-be assassin of President Reagan, now resides. Rouse, one of these men, realized after seven years of confinement in the John Howard Pavilion that his lawyer had not cut a good deal for him.[35] The crime he committed carried a maximum sentence of one year. Furthermore, he was getting no meaningful treatment, and without a cure he would never be released. His lawyers took his complaint to Judge Bazelon, who ruled that Rouse had a right to treatment. And Judge Bazelon had the gall to tell the psychiatrists at St. Elizabeth's something about treatment. Like the person who sees that the Emperor has no clothes, Judge Bazelon told the psychiatrists that mere confinement in the John Howard Pavilion did not constitute milieu therapy.[36] There is a difference between being locked up and being a member of Maxwell Jones' therapeutic community. At any rate, Rouse, who was subjected to quasi-criminal confinement, gave rise to the right to treatment. Judges would later go much further in telling psychiatrists how to treat their patients, and when the psychiatrists balked, psychologists, social workers, and nurses were authorized as legitimate substitutes by the courts.[37]

Next came the famous right to refuse treatment. It began in California, where a psychiatrist devised a radical form of aversive conditioning. Mentally ill offenders who repeatedly harmed themselves or others were seized by the staff, held down, and immediately given injections of succinylcholine. This is the curare-like drug used to control convulsions during electroconvulsive therapy. In preparation for electroconvulsive therapy, the patient is anesthetized, intubated, given succinylcholine, and then ventilated because breathing is paralyzed by succinylcholine. When given to an unanesthetized patient, or should I say victim, it creates a feeling of suffocating to death, because in fact the victim is actually suffocating. This aversive experience was intended to be therapeutic and to control violence to self and others. Another such aversive procedure involved administering apomorphine to produce vomiting. But federal judges confronted with these stories concluded that not everything psychiatrists did was treatment and that a court might consider some of the things psychiatrists do to patients cruel and unusual punishment, a violation of the Eighth Amendment to our Constitution.[38] The most publicized right to refuse treatment case, however, occurred in Michigan, where doctors attempting to pursue the work of Mark and Ervine set up an experimental protocol to make microscopic lesions in the amygdala of supposedly sexually violent patients. They intended to compare the results with a similar group given Depo-Provera (medroxyprogesterone), a drug related to the female hormone progesterone. The patients to be thus treated had been placed in quasi-criminal confinement as sexual psychopaths. Only one subject was found for this experiment. He preferred brain surgery to Depo-Provera, but the procedure never took place. Instead, this situation resulted in the famous anti-psychosurgery lawsuit, *Kaimowitz v. Department of Mental Health.*[39] The case held that patients had constitutional rights, including First Amendment rights, protecting them against such treatment.

From succinylcholine, apomorphine, and psychosurgery of quasi-criminal patient-inmates grew the constitutional right to refuse treatment, a right which is now being extended to such ordinary treatments as neuroleptics for psychotics in all mental hospitals. My thesis, briefly illustrated by these examples, is that the current legal regulation of American psychiatry began in quasi-criminal institutions, and those legal precedents were then extended to ordinary mental hospitals. Those quasi-criminal institutions had their origins in the minds of forensic psychiatrists and other progressives who attempted to help the criminal justice system deal with violence by making it a sickness.

This chapter in American law and psychiatry, the quasi-criminal institution, is coming to an end. The recent model legal standards of the American Bar Association call for the repeal of all "statutes which provided for special sentencing and treatment of quasi-criminal offenders."[40] But in the meantime, in the United States some unfortunate things have happened. The attack on psychiatry, although begun in the quasi-criminal setting, has had its greatest impact on public mental hospitals. Disenchanted with psychiatry for a variety of reasons that have little to do with the failures of quasi-criminal confinement, lawmakers effected radical reforms of the laws of civil commitment. Mental illness and the need for treatment alone was rejected as a justification for involuntary treatment. The courts increasingly required that the alleged patient be mentally ill and dangerous. With such laws controlling involuntary admission, the patient population of public mental hospitals has increasingly begun to resemble the population once confined in quasi-criminal facilities. Some psychiatrists in America have written about a new class of chronic mental patients, males between age 20 and 40, who move back and forth between prisons and mental hospitals, who have serious character disorders bordering on schizophrenia, who are more violent, and who are resistant to neuroleptic treatment. This group may indeed represent a new class of mental patients. On the other hand, they may reflect legal reforms under which judges and not doctors "label" the mentally ill. It is ironic that a legal system which has recognized and criticized psychiatry because of its inability to predict and its failure to treat dangerous persons in quasi-criminal confinement would make that very function psychiatry's principal responsibility in public mental hospitals. And now, having given us a responsibility we cannot competently fulfill, they sue us for malpractice when our patients are violent. That is the tortured path of legal progress in the United States.

LESSONS FOR THE FUTURE

What are the lessons to be learned from the failures of the Criminal Justice System and the failures of psychiatry in its attempts to help the Criminal Justice System? The first lesson is that the problems of the Criminal Justice System are massive. Psychiatry is not to blame for this, and lawyers and judges who attack psychiatry as though it had caused the mess are looking at the pimple on the nose and not at the congestive heart failure. It is time to draw clear lines. The Criminal Justice System, whatever its problems, must be responsible for protecting society. And psychiatry must be responsible for treating the mentally ill. Only when violence is a symptom of a treatable mental illness should psychiatry be involved. These basic guidelines should control all future policy and legislation. This does not mean that psychiatrists should not work in prisons, it means that they should not be in control of prisons.

The second lesson is that therapeutic optimism about the treatment of violence has gotten psychiatry into trouble. I mentioned at the outset of this essay the supposed role that limbic system disorder plays in violence. If I can count as an objective observer, it seems to me that the importance of this disease of the brain was much exaggerated by Mark and Ervine. Does anyone now seriously believe that it explains a substantial portion of violent crime, or that drugs or psychosurgery will cure the kinds of violence I have described? And even if Freud and Menninger are correct about the evils of human nature, is there anyone who seriously believes that psychoanalysis or psychodynamic therapy is a realistic remedy for violence, or that psychiatry of any kind has a cure for racism, economic inequality, and the many discontents of civilization? Does anyone seriously believe that psychiatry has a cure for the five murders a day in New York City? Nothing I have said is meant to suggest that I am opposed to psychiatric research on violence, be it research on the brain or on the mind. It is the task of the medical scientist to chip away at these problems. Nor am I opposed to attempts by psychiatrists to help violent patients who want to be helped. Physicians have always tried to help even when the available treatments were grossly inadequate. What I have been attacking in this essay are the giant leaps from chipping away at a problem to major legal reforms, the leap from trying to help to forcing people to submit to our help because they are violent. And I must add one further criticism. The four paradigms of modern psychiatric theory—biological, behavioral, psychodynamic, and social—can each generate one or more theories of violence. But all of those theories will in the end share a common failing. They are all anchored in some form of determinism, they all make violence into a disease, and thus our theories undermine the contemporary person's sense of moral responsibility for violence. I have already described to you how the Criminal Justice System in its own way undermines the sense of moral responsibility. We too have undermined moral responsibility with our deterministic theories of violence. Psychiatry belongs to a family of disciplines which combine the sciences and the humanities. It is a discipline, therefore, that need not be at odds with law. Law itself is a member of our family. Both law and psychiatry must begin a basic rebuilding process, and moral responsibility for violence must be part of both blueprints for the future.

REFERENCES

1. *Ne v York Times*, March 31, 1980.

2. *Kerner Report on Civil Disorders, Supplemental Studies for the National Advisory Commission on Civil Disorders* (Praeger, 1968).

3. National Safety Council, *Accident Facts* (1982).

4. B. Bettelheim, *Freud and Man's Soul* (A. Knopf, distributed by Random House, 1983).

5. S. Freud, *Civilization and Its Discontents* (W.W. Norton and Co., 1962).

6. Mark, Sweet, and Ervin, Role of Brain Disease in Riots and Urban Violence, *Journal of the American Medical Association*, Vol. 201, p. 895 (1967).

7. V. Mark and F. Ervin, *Violence and the Brain* (Harper and Row, 1970).

8. *Ibid.*, p. 1.

9. Department of Justice, *Crime in the United States* (1982).

10. Wolfgang and Tracey, The 1945 and 1958 Birth Cohorts: A Comparison of the Prevalence, Incidence and Severity of Delinquent Behavior (unpublished paper, University of Pennsylvania, 1982).

11. Personal Communication, Professor Alan Dershowitz.

12. *See* W. Spelman, The Crime Control Effectiveness of Selective Incapacitation Policies (included in M. Moore, S. Estrich, and D. McGillis, *Dealing with Dangerous Offenders* (unpublished paper, Harvard, 1983).

13. P. Greenwood and A. Abrahamse, *Selective Incapacitation* (Rand Corporation, 1982).

14. *Ibid.*

15. M. Moore, S. Estrich, and D. McGillis, *op. cit.*

16. *Ibid.*

17. Greenwood and Abrahamse, *Op. cit.* note 13 and M.A. Peterson, H.B. Braiker, and S.M. Polich, *Who Commits Crimes: A Survey of Prison Inmates* (Oegeschlager, Gunn, and Hain, 1981).

18. Wolfgang and Tracey, *Op. cit.* note 10.

19. Note, Selective Incapacitation: Reducing Crime Through Predictions of Recidivism, *Harvard Law Review*, Vol. 96, p. 511 (1982).

20. *See* D. Stone, Selective Incapacitation and Career Criminal Programs: An In Depth Analysis (unpublished paper, Harvard Law School, 1983).

21. *New York Times*, January 4, 1981.

22. *Ibid.*

23. Vera Institute of Justice, *Felony Arrests: Their Prosecution and Disposition in New York City's Courts* (1977).

24. A. Dershowitz, *The Best Defense* (Random House, 1982).

25. U.S. Bureau of Justice, *Parole in the United States* (Annual, 1977-to date).

26. *Ibid.*

27. J. Petersilia, *Racial Disparities in the Criminal Justice System* (Rand Corporation, 1983).

28. *See* A. Cohen, G. Cole, and R. Bailey, *Prison Violence* (Lexington Books, 1976); A Scacco Jr., *Rape in Prison* (Charles C Thomas, 1975).

29. *See, United States v. Bailey*, 100 S.Ct. 624 (1980).

30. *See, Graddick v. Newman*, 453 U.S. 928 (1981).

31. *Op. cit.* note 9.

32. A. Stone, *Mental Health and Law: A System in Transition* (National Institute of Mental Health, 1975).

33. Maryland Annotated Code Art. 31B §§1-19 (1967) (adopted 1951).

34. *Op. cit.* note 32.

35. *Rouse v. Cameron*, 373 F.2d 451 (D.C. Cir. 1966).

36. *Ibid.*

37. *Wyatt v. Stickney*, 344 F. Supp. 373 (M.D. Ala. 1972).

38. *See Mackey v. Procunier*, 477 F.2d 877 (9th Cir. 1973); *Knecht v. Gillman*, 488 F.2d 1136 (8th Cir. 1973).

39. *Kaimowitz v. Department of Mental Health*, Civil #73-19434-AW (Cir. Ct. Wayne County, Mich., July 10, 1973).

40. American Bar Association, *Criminal Justice Mental Health Standards* (Tentative Draft, July 1983).

III

The Ethics of Forensic Psychiatry:
A View from the Ivory Tower

A T A RECENT MEETING of sixty federal judges from around the country, one of the trial judges defined the essence of the distinction between trial and appellate judges. "Trial judges," he said, "are in the front lines of legal warfare, they are foot soldiers involved in bloody hand-to-hand combat. Appellate judges, in contrast, sit on a safe hill overlooking the battlefield. When the fighting is over, the appellate judge comes down from his position of safety and goes about shooting the wounded." Similarly one could describe forensic psychiatry as a kind of hand-to-hand combat, and now as never before, the troops are wounded and bloody. Scholarly criticism has been blistering,[1] and after the trial of John Hinckley, the media have been unrelenting in their attacks. Now, when forensic psychiatrists need encouragement, healing balms, and soothing treatment, I have come down from my ivory tower to "shoot the wounded."

But forensic psychiatrists need not be afraid: like the trial judges, they will survive to fight again. In fact, though wounded and bloody they are paradoxically stronger than ever before. The legal assault on psychiatry of the past two decades had one consistent result. It took discretionary authority away from the psychiatrist and handed it over to the courts. But the courts, in order to take on this burden responsibly, require more, not less psychiatric testimony. The more they distrust forensic psychiatrists, the more they need them. Whatever the reasons, forensic psychiatry though condemned and repudiated seems nonetheless to be flourishing. There is an array of related journals,[2] new organizations and subspecialty boards, a remarkable number of well-trained competent practitioners, and an increasingly sophisticated intellectual dialogue. In a stagnant psychiatric economy, forensic psychiatry is one of the few growth stocks. The sudden boom in forensic psychology gives further evidence of the strength and attractiveness of the market.

Although I have spent the past 20 years teaching, studying, and writing about Law and Psychiatry, I am not a forensic psychiatrist. The reasons why I am not are in fact what I shall here discuss. What has kept me out of the courtroom is my concern about the ambiguity of the intellectual and ethical boundaries of forensic psychiatry. At the outset, let me state what I think the boundary problems are.

First, there is the basic boundary question. Does psychiatry have anything true to say to which the courts should listen?

Second, there is the risk that the forensic psychiatrist will go too far and twist the rules of justice and fairness to help the patient.

Third, there is the opposite risk that the forensic psychiatrist will deceive the patient in order to serve justice and fairness.

Fourth, there is the danger that forensic psychiatrists will prostitute the profession, as they are alternately seduced and assaulted by the power of the adversarial system.*

Finally, as one struggles with these four issues (Does one have something true to say? Is one twisting justice? Is one deceiving the patient? Is one prostituting the profession?), there is the additional problem that forensic psychiatrists seem to be without any clear guidelines as to what is proper and ethical. In this regard I shall be commenting on (1) the good clinical practice standard, (2) the scientific standard, (3) the truth and honesty standard, and (4) the adversary

---

* Different problems arise when the psychiatrist testifies as *amicus* to the court. Although many psychiatrists prefer this role, it is, from the point of view of Anglo-American law, employing the procedures of the inquisitional process. The difficulties in making inquisitional exceptions to the adversarial process go far beyond the scope of this essay, and indeed of psychiatric testimony. The use of psychiatric testimony in the inquisitional framework is discussed in the first chapter, which examines political misuse of psychiatry.

standard. For now I shall simply assert that the American Medical Association's *Principles of Ethics with Annotations for Psychiatrists*[3] are irrelevant as guidelines for forensic psychiatrists. Eventually, I shall test this proposition by examining the ethical complaints that have been voiced against forensic testimony for the prosecution as considered by the Supreme Court in the *Barefoot v. Estelle*[4] case. I will argue that there is no neutral general principle by which such testimony can be called unethical.

PSYCHIATRY AND TRUTH

The most basic question is whether psychiatrists have true answers to the legal and moral questions posed by the law. Immanuel Kant, who after two centuries is still a dominant figure in the landscape of moral philosophy, had strong opinions about this question. He wrote, "con-cerning the question whether the mental condition of the agent was one of derangement or of a fixed purpose held with a sound understanding, forensic medicine is meddling with alien business."[5] Kant would give a different meaning to the ancient designation of the forensic psychiatrist as an *alienist*. Kant also wrote, "physicians are generally still not advanced enough to see deeply into the mechanisms inside a human being in order to determine the cause of an unnatural transgression of the moral law."[6]

Kant's opinion was both that our science was inadequate and that as to moral questions, alienists were meddling in alien business. A century later, Freud echoed Kant's sentiments in a new vocabulary: "[T]he physician will leave it to the jurist to construct for social purposes a responsibility that is artificially limited to the metapsycholog-ical ego."[7] Since Freud's time some psychoanalysts have attempted to generate a theory of moral responsibility not limited to the metapsy-chological ego. But Freud's most authoritative interpreter—certainly his most orthodox—Heinz Hartmann, in his monograph *Psychoanalysis and Moral Values*,[8] drew a sharp clear line: psychoanalysis could say something about why people come to hold the values and morality they hold but could say nothing substantive about those values and morals.

This purist position of Kant-Freud-Hartmann would suggest that even today the forensic psychiatrist outside the therapeutic context is meddling in alien business. Given the basic premise of these purists, the attempt to delineate the ethical boundaries of forensic psychiatry is vacuous. Psychiatrists are immediately over the boundary when they go

from psychiatry to law. To ask what are the ethical boundaries for this
practice would be rather like asking what are the ethical boundaries for
an imposter. From this purist perspective the problem with forensic
psychiatry is not the adversarial process and its use of adversarial
experts, which distorts the "science." Rather purists think it is as
absurd for psychiatrists to decide legal-moral questions and questions of
social justice as neutral scientific friends of the court as it is for them to
be adversarial witnesses.

The purist position can be reached by different kinds of reasoning.
Intellectually, there seem to be five strands that make up the purist
position. I shall briefly allude to them and suggest their relevance to
forensic psychiatry.

THE INTELLECTUAL CHASM

First, there is the problem of the fact-value distinction. This is the
philosophical line followed by Hartmann. It assumes that there is a
sharp distinction between facts in the objective sphere of science and
values in the subjective sphere of morality and law and that the gap
between them is unbridgeable. The purist sees forensic psychiatrists as
simply confusing the two spheres or as failing to recognize their
distinctions. Forensic psychiatrists present their values as though they
were scientific facts.

Two lines have been taken here. One is Hartmann's, and according
to it the psychoanalyst has nothing to say about moral questions, except
possibly to explain how people come to hold their particular moral
values, and that is the end of the matter. The second line says that
psychoanalysts should acknowledge their own value preferences—for
example, a belief that our society should place the interests of children
above those of adults—and then in light of the psychoanalytic facts
develop particular legal policies. This is the familiar strategy adopted by
Goldstein, Freud, and Solnit in formulating a variety of legal rules
having to do with the interests of children.[9] Since such views have had
considerable acceptance and influence, they merit more detailed, though
still too brief, consideration among the five strands of the purist
position.

When one looks at what these authors offer as psychoanalytic facts,
one must question whether the purported facts are not themselves
tainted by value judgments. Goldstein, Freud, and Solnit offer as a

psychoanalytic fact the claim that events affecting young children are more important than those affecting older children.

Children, in this conception, are like a biological system. When exposed to a trauma at an early point they are more apt to be harmed than when trauma happens at a later date. This is the implicit assumption behind the authors' psychoanalytic "fact," and although the analogy is intuitively appealing, it is in essence unwarranted biological reduction-ism—unwarranted by empirical observation and by psychoanalytic theory itself. This implicit biological reductionism creates the illusion that the authors are talking about facts rather than values.

They argue, for example, that given their explicit value preference for children over adults and given these psychoanalytic facts, the law should keep a small child with his psychological parents rather than make him suffer the separation trauma inherent in handing him over to his biological parents—even if at a later time the decision to deprive him of his biological parents may be troubling. But in fact the empirical studies of separation trauma have to do with the unreplaced loss of the psychological parent, not transfer to a biological parent who is eager to become a psychological parent—a transfer in which the psychological parent could assist under the best circumstances.

Even if there were empirical evidence that the trauma of such transfer is apparent in the short run, there is no evidence that in the long run the trauma of transfer is worse than the trauma of deprivation of one's biological parents. The latter depends on a multitude of variables, including the meaning of the transfer and the meaning of having biological parents.[10] The issue of meaning suggests the fallacy in their reductionistic concept of trauma.

Trauma in psychoanalysis is psychic trauma. Psychic trauma involves an interactive event plus its meaning and its conscious and unconscious significance. Indeed, the meaning and significance of an observable event over time may well determine whether that event was a trauma or a helpful emotional experience. Whether or not these criticisms are entirely correct, they show the perils of trying to separate facts and values, even when those making the claim are acutely aware of the difficulty. Indeed it is possible to argue that Goldstein, Freud, and Solnit can best be understood as having a value preference not for children, but for adults who devote themselves to children, that is, psychological parents. One can argue about the pros and cons of such a value preference, but one should not claim it is an argument about psychoanalytic facts.

The second problem area is that of free will vs. determinism. The debate has never been resolved by psychiatrists. It is relevant to every question of volition and responsibility. It is a principal theme in Professor Morse's lengthy and detailed attack on the fallacies of psychodynamic testimony in criminal trials.[11] Without a resolution of the problem it is impossible to evaluate the significance of the psychia-trist's testimony. If his account of a party's condition is presented in terms of deterministic causal forces which preclude the party's being responsible for his own actions, then we may draw one conclusion.

If the account is one which outlines deterministic causes which somehow leave untouched a sphere of free will (as Kant might have said), one need not draw the same conclusion. If the psychiatric account should be understood as something other than a deterministic causal account, its implications could again be different.

A third area is the deconstruction of the self: without the unity of the self, moral reasoning becomes impossible. It is the deepest, most basic theoretical dilemma of modern psychiatry, and it is not just the work of psychoanalysis and the metapsychological ego. It is an issue in behavioral and biological psychiatry. It is specifically relevant to claims about how the criminal law should deal with multiple personality, dissociative reactions, and unconscious forces in general.

Without an understanding of when the self retains its unity and how that unity is essential to moral conduct, we cannot assess the relevance of psychiatric accounts for moral-legal questions concerning how the law should deal with the party to whom the psychiatric accounts apply. Freud implicitly acknowledged this problem when he wrote about "a responsibility that is artificially limited to the metapsy-chological ego." The moral theorist would argue that Freud "artifi-cially" divided the self into the ego, the superego, and the id. But this deconstruction of the self is characteristic of modern thought. The self, like Humpty Dumpty, has been shattered, and all the king's philoso-phers and all the king's lawyers cannot put Humpty Dumpty together again.

The fourth area is the mind-brain problem.[12] The mind-brain problem plagues all our endeavors to account for human actions. It is particularly pertinent to alcoholism, to drug abuse, and to recent theories of violence. Whatever understanding science may offer of the nature and functions of the brain, we cannot assess its relevance to the law's proper disposition of a particular party's case without taking a position on the mind-brain problem. If mental states are somehow reducible to brain states, then scientific accounts of the brain could in principle provide full accounts of human psychology. But on any other hypothesis about the mind-brain problem, the very relevance of information about the brain is less clear. If there is somehow a mind-brain interaction, its relevance depends on the nature of that interaction; if there is minimal or no mind-brain interaction, its relevance is minimal or nonexistent. If this is too abstract, think of the *Torsney*[13] case in which a white police officer's unprovoked killing of a black youth was attributed to temporal lobe epilepsy resulting in a verdict of not guilty by reason of insanity. The next chapter will offer examples from the Hinckley trial, and the reader will see how important the mind-brain problem is to forensic psychiatry. Professor Michael Moore has demonstrated, to my satisfaction, that America's most influential forensic psychiatrist, Isaac Ray, got lost in the mind-brain trap and never got out.[14]

Last, there is the chasm that has opened up between what Kuhn[15] would call "normal science," and morality—a chasm which characterizes almost all of modern thought and, particularly, behavioral sciences. The chasm can be seen in terms of some of the preceding strands. Science is the realm of fact, while morality is the realm of value, so that the gap between fact and value contributes to the distance between science and morality. Similarly, science is the attempt to discover causal explanations of behavior, while morality may seem to presuppose the absence of such explanations of behavior.

The apparent incompatibility of free will and determinism thus further splits science and morality. Finally, science, particularly "bench science," seems to be well equipped to study the brain, but it cannot apply its methods directly to the study of the mind. The mind is an essential aspect of the domain where morality has its more ready application. The mind-brain question thus also contributes to the chasm between morality and normal science. It is that chasm which forensic psychiatry tries to bridge. I shall touch on some of these strands, but here let me say only that the purist position is not easily dismissed—it raises serious questions about the basic legitimacy of forensic psychiatry.

Each forensic psychiatrist may have resolved the five intellectual problems in his or her own mind, but I doubt that any of us would claim that forensic psychiatry has achieved a consensus on these issues. Philosophers[16] and lawyers[17] might also claim to have resolved these questions, but it seems that they have no more consensus as to these problems than do psychiatrists. The conceptual problems which have been outlined are not limited to psychodynamic testimony. They apply equally to behavioral, biological, and social psychiatry. They apply even to what many would consider the hard science part of psychiatry.

THE GOOD CLINICAL PRACTICE STANDARD

Now it can be argued against my position that all that I have said is ap' plicable to everything psychiatrists do and not just to forensic psychia' try. This counterargument leads to the good clinical practice standard, the argument made by my colleague and friend, Andrew Watson. He believes that psychiatrists are constantly making value judgments and expressing moral convictions implicitly, if not explicitly. He would acknowledge all of the difficult intellectual problems I have enumerated, but he would say they are just as relevant to clinical practice as to forensic psychiatry. Finally, he would say, if we do it in our office why can't we do it in the courtroom? We even make predictions about future dangerousness in our office. Do we believe in the practice of psychiatry or don't we? I shall accept Doctor Watson's "good clinical practice" argument so that we can cross the first boundary into the law.

But I shall first take you back almost two centuries to enter the courtroom. From this safe vantage point we can consider twisting justice, deceiving the patient, and prostituting the profession. Let me quote the interrogation of a "forensic" psychiatrist that took place in 1801. It is reported by Nigel Walker in his treatise on crime and insanity in England[18] The trial involved a Jew who had been caught stealing spoons.

The Jews of the London community had set up a society for visiting the sick and doing charitable deeds. The society employed a Doctor Leo, who three times testified at the Old Bailey on behalf of his Jewish patients. On all three occasions, his patients had been accused of shoplifting. This was his third appearance. First Doctor Leo was questioned by the court.

Court: Are you particularly versed in this disorder of the human mind?
Leo: I am.
Court: Then you are what is called a mad doctor? [Walker adds, "no doubt there was laughter in the court at this sally."]

Then he was cross examined by the prosecutor.

The Prosecutor: Have you ever given evidence before?

Leo: [Walker adds, "almost losing his temper."] I believe that I have. Is that any matter of consequence?

The Prosecutor: Upon your oath, have you or have you not been examined as a witness here before?

Leo: I never took any notice.

The Prosecutor: Have you not been here twice?

Leo: Yes.

Prosecutor: Have you not been here more than three times?

Leo: I cannot say.

Prosecutor: Have you not been here before as a witness and a Jew physician, to give an account of a prisoner as a madman, to get him off upon the ground of insanity?

The nastiness with which Doctor Leo was treated by these English contemporaries of Immanuel Kant (who shared their anti-Semitism) cannot be attributed to their intellectual position, but their examination of the witness strikes two notes which resonate even today in the halls of Congress and our state legislatures—namely, that the psychiatrist is a bad joke in the courtroom, and that forensic psychiatrists are there to get defendants off.[19]

The question I would pose to Doctor Watson is, what could he say today in defense of Doctor Leo's testimony? He could tell the prosecutor as I would that anti-Semitism is vile and repugnant, particularly so in an officer of the court. But could he argue, given the primitive state of psychiatry in 1801, that Doctor Leo had a good clinical understanding of what he called "the mania" of his patient for stealing spoons? Could he say that his purpose in testifying was other than to help a fellow Jew escape what the law of the day considered just punishment? Was he not twisting justice and fairness to help his patient and prostituting his profession to do so?

Doctor Watson might say that my example is ridiculous and far fetched, but I ask him and those who share his views to imagine some psychiatric historian two hundred years from now examining the good clinical practice and the clinical diagnostic concepts advanced by the psychiatrists on either side of the Hinckley trial. Is there much chance that the historian of our profession would conclude that those psychiatrists, to use Kant's language, "saw deeply into the mechanisms inside the human being in order to determine the cause of an unnatural transgression of the moral law"?[20] Or would the historian more likely comment on the primitive state of clinical psychiatry in 1982: its incomplete understanding of the brain and the mind and its bizarre diagnostic categories as set out in DSM-III?

THE SCIENTIFIC STANDARD

Another of my friends and colleagues, Loren Roth, is of the view that what should guide ethical forensic psychiatrists is their commitment to the standards of science. As I understand his view, he wants to set a higher standard than Andrew Watson's "good clinical judgment." I think Loren Roth shares my view that "good clinical judgment" is a precariously egocentric standard.

I once assisted in some empirical research on humor. It turned out that every subject I gave the "Mirth Response Test" to thought he or she had a very good sense of humor.[21] Similarly, it seems to me that every psychiatrist thinks he has very good clinical judgment. Doctor Roth wants to find a brighter line. He would limit his testimony to what he knows to be scientific. Based on that standard, he would not allow forensic psychiatrists to answer ultimate legal questions which have no scientific answers. But I would claim that if forensic psychiatrists limited themselves to the standards of bench scientists, not only would they not testify about ultimate legal questions; their lips would be sealed in the courtroom.

Psychiatry is still closer to social science than to physical science, and Max Weber's statement about social science applies to us. We must expect that what we believe to be right will soon be proved wrong.[22] It is no disgrace to work at a primitive science. As Jonas Rappeport asks, "Are we embarrassed to let the public know that the state of our art is such that we do not know everything and that there are different schools and theories in psychiatry?"[23] The hubris in psychiatry has come from passing it off as scientific certainty or claiming that we know things beyond a reasonable doubt. But if psychiatry is an art, as Rappeport's candor suggests, how do we adhere to Roth's standards of science?

The relevant difference between clinical practice and forensic practice has sometimes been discussed under the heading of the psychiatrist as a double agent. I do not want to rehearse that discussion, although it is a valuable way to analyze these problems. A forensic examination for the other side confronts the psychiatrist with problems of being a double agent—problems which otherwise often go unnoticed.

Rappeport's solution to the thorny dilemma of examining a patient for the other side is for the interviewer to recognize the potential for abuses of confidentiality and always to inform the patient which side he or she is serving.[24] But I agree with Seymour Halleck that informing the examinee of the fact that you are a double agent is necessary but not sufficient to resolve the conflict of interests. There are two reasons for this conclusion; I put off one until my discussion of testimony in capital punishment. Skilled interviewers like Doctors Halleck, Roth, and Watson will create a relationship in which the examinee can readily forget that he has been warned. It is no accident that good clinicians are often emotionally seductive human beings who inspire personal trust. Emotionally seducing a schizophrenic to reach him in his autistic withdrawal may or may not be bad technique, but it is certainly easier to justify as a parameter of treatment than as a method of obtaining information to determine whether he should have visitation rights with his children.

THE ETHICAL DIALECTIC OF PSYCHIATRY

The crucial word for me in what I have just said is "justify": when our goal as psychiatrists is to do our best to ease a patient's suffering, we have a powerful justification. It is the justification for every physician who did not wait for science and theory to be perfected. Do whatever you can to help your patient and *primum nil nocere*, first of all do no harm.[25] These contradictory claims constitute the ethical dialectic of the physician's practice. We have not yet found the synthesis of this thesis and antithesis; our fate is to struggle within this contradiction. But as physicians treating patients, we know what the ethical struggle is. We know the boundaries of the ethical debate. When we turn our skills to forensic psychiatry, when we serve the system of justice, we can no longer agree on the boundaries of the debate.

A few words about the adversary system and how it bears on this ethical dialectic. Let me return to Doctor Leo at the Old Bailey in 1801. Doctor Leo is typical of a certain kind of psychiatrist who goes to court: the psychiatrist who knows very little about the law but who goes to court out of sympathy for a client or for a cause. To some forensic psychiatrists these are the real villains, the amateurs who do not recognize that forensic psychiatry is a professional subspecialty.

But it is not the amateur's naïveté about the law which interests me; rather, it is his impulse to help the patient or to serve some cause which the patient represents. The amateur, it seems to me, is still trying to act according to the basic ethical calling of the physician—he is trying to relieve suffering, he is still struggling within the ethical dialectic of the healer.

It is my impression that this impulse has not been limited to amateurs. Many distinguished forensic psychiatrists have felt more comfortable acting on behalf of criminal defendants than on behalf of the prosecution. The current professional attitude of forensic psychiatry is to provide testimony for both sides, in part because otherwise the forensic psychiatrist runs the risk of being pilloried by the prosecution as a defense-biased witness. But it seems to me there has long been a very comfortable ideological fit between being a forensic psychiatrist and being against capital punishment, being therapeutic rather than puni- tive, being against the prosecution and what was seen as the harsh status quo in criminal law. This ideological fit has begun to come apart in recent history. But during the days when Judge David Bazelon and American psychiatry had their love affair the fit was real. Those were the halcyon days when the concept of treatment and the concept of social justice were virtually indistinguishable.

Here we confront what I believe is still a lingering confusion in the enterprise of forensic psychiatry. The problem is that helping the patient—which is the ethical thesis of the practitioner—becomes the ethical temptation in the legal context. What principle does the forensic psychiatrist have to restrain himself against this temptation? What is his equivalent to the therapist's antithesis of do no harm, particularly when he is cajoled by the lawyers, dazzled by the media spotlight, and paid more than Blue Cross/Blue Shield? I have already suggested that I believe Doctor Watson's good clinical practice is a precariously egocen- tric standard for self-administered ethical restraints. One only needs to hear forensic psychiatrists criticizing each other's ethics to see how precarious it is. Doctor Roth's scientific standard would, in my opinion, lead to a vow of silence.

THE STANDARD OF TRUTH

My colleague and friend, Paul Applebaum, has suggested that the standard of truth should govern the forensic psychiatrist. In a moral dialogue it seems to me that this is a very appealing standard, but like Kant's categorical imperative it is much more convincing as an abstract statement than it is useful as a practical guide to conduct. I assume that Paul Applebaum's standard of the truth is not the same as the one I raised at the beginning of this chapter—the truth in some absolute sense. That kind of absolute truth keeps the psychiatrists out of the courtroom. What Doctor Applebaum means, I think, is closer to honesty; the forensic psychiatrist must honestly believe what he says and should not allow his views to be distorted by the media spotlight, by the lawyers, or by the money. He should be an honest, good clinical practitioner. Let us consider how this standard fares in the adversarial context.[26]

The adversarial system, of course, requires psychiatrists for both sides. That was one of the complaints against the old lineup of concerned psychiatrists for the defense: psychiatry was not being fair to the adversarial system. My late friend and colleague Seymour Pollack was particularly concerned about this issue,[27] and even Judge Bazelon lamented the lack of competent psychiatrists on both sides. Bazelon wanted psychiatrists to recognize and accede to the higher ethical framework of the adversarial system's search for justice.[28] The problem he failed to consider was how the psychiatrists would square the ethical imperative of the healing profession with the adversarial goals of criminal prosecution.

TESTIFYING FOR THE PROSECUTION IN CAPITAL PUNISHMENT

To illuminate that problem I want to examine what I take to be the most challenging case—Doctor Grigson's practice of testifying for the prosecution in capital punishment cases, such as *Barefoot v. Estelle*. At the outset, let me say that I disagree with those who would claim that such testimony is unethical.[29] By that I mean it does not violate the American Psychiatric Association's canons of ethics as I would interpret them, it does not violate the good clinical practice standard, and it does not violate the truth as honesty standard. It may violate Doctor Roth's scientific standard, but again I claim that almost everything but a vow of silence would violate his standard.

The practice in question is as follows. The defendant had been found guilty of a capital offense. The court then heard testimony from Doctor Grigson, who had never personally examined the defendant. (A prior decision by the Supreme Court had dealt with an earlier practice in which psychiatrists who had examined defendants for some other purpose then testified against them at this capital punishment stage.[30] This decision is discussed at length in other chapters.) Here, there had been no prior professional contact and therefore no possible allegation could be made that Doctor Grigson had violated the rights of the defendant. Doctor Grigson was asked a series of hypothetical questions relevant to the defendant's history and criminal behavior. His answers, expressed with almost absolute clinical conviction, were that such persons are sociopaths: they are and will be very dangerous, and they do not experience remorse. Dangerousness and lack of remorse are two of the criteria which are relevant to the death penalty.

Now what is unethical about such testimony? I assume that Doctor Grigson believes what he is saying. One certainly has no basis to assume otherwise just because he almost always testifies for the prosecu- tion, and in favor of the death penalty. I assume he is as honest and sin- cere and as much committed to the good clinical practice standard as the forensic psychiatrists who almost always testify against the death penalty or who go around the country urging verdicts of not guilty by reason of insanity.

After all, Doctor Grigson and the other psychiatrists testify under oath; they are sworn to tell the truth. "You do solemnly swear to testify to the truth, the whole truth, and nothing but the truth. So help you God."[31] I may not have done justice to Doctor Applebaum's standard— he may have been thinking along different lines (I shall return to this matter of sworn testimony). But if I have made my friends into straw- men, it was to make clear to you that my ideas are part of an intellectual dialogue with them.

Let me turn briefly and finally to examine Doctor Grigson's testimony in light of the APA's own Principles of Ethics. Here the language is specific. What annotations could one cite if one wished to make an ethical complaint against such testimony in capital punishment cases? One might allege that he gave diagnostic opinions about a patient he never examined.

The relevant annotation, annotation 3 of section 7, clearly is not aimed at courtroom testimony. It was added by the APA after the Goldwater fiasco.[32] Hundreds of psychiatrists were willing to fill out questionnaires and diagnose Barry Goldwater as mentally ill during the Presidential elections of 1964. The incident, which says something about the fact-value problem in psychiatry, embarrassed the psychiatric establishment, resulting in the addition of this annotation. I opposed this change at the time as a denial of free speech and of every psychiatrist's God-given right to make a fool of himself. If the psychi- atric establishment banned everything that embarrassed them, they would ban forensic psychiatry. And if annotation 3 of section 7 were strictly enforced, forensic psychiatrists could never write or lecture relying on decided case law and the trial transcripts which present relevant clinical aspects of "patients" like Hinckley, Sirhan, Poddar, Torsney, etcetera. Parts of this very book would be unethical.

Furthermore, if Doctor Grigson violated annotation 3 then it is also regularly violated when forensic psychiatrists routinely answer hypothetical questions about testamentary capacity long after a person they never examined has died.

Testifying to hypothetical questions in court is not unethical, at least as I interpret the language and the history of annotation 3 of section 7. The procedure is used by Doctor Grigson, of course, to escape the double agent conflict I mentioned earlier. Never having examined the patient, there is no doctor-patient relation, no false expectation, no deception, and no conflict of interest.

To object to Doctor Grigson's procedure is to attempt to deprive the prosecution of a legitimate adversarial witness. Forensic psychiatry has no general neutral principle for doing that. We have the intuition that such testimony in death penalty cases is unethical because of our basic practical ethical guideline to do all we can to ease the suffering of our patients. Ironically, this basic guideline is no longer part of the American Medical Association's ethical guidelines—nor is "first of all do no harm." If we were to take this basic guideline very seriously, how could we ever be zealous advocates for the prosecution in death penalty cases? And if the legal system thought we were bound by this practical ethical guideline, how could we serve the adversarial system of criminal justice? The Supreme Court seems to share these views. It upheld the constitutionality of Doctor Grigson's hypothetical testimony despite a dissenting opinion that raised the ethical questions.[33] If there are problems with Doctor Grigson's testimony, as I believe there are and as I shall try to demonstrate in later chapters, the fault lies not in his professional integrity but in forensic psychiatry.

THE APPEAL TO NONMEDICAL VALUES

When we object to the ethical conduct of Doctor Grigson as the prosecution's expert, it is because we want to have our cake and eat it too. We want to be doctors who are healers and we want to serve the adversary system. My colleague and friend, Laurence Tancredi, has commented that to many moral philosophers, justice is itself a beneficence. He is certainly correct, but justice is a beneficence to a society of unidentified persons—that is, to the general good. In contrast, the doctor's practical ethical duty is to ease the suffering of particular identified patients. Medicine has not yet solved the problem of how to balance the particular good of the identified patient against the general good of the unidentified masses. We lose our practical ethical guidelines when we try to serve such greater good in the courtroom.

Consider in this regard the Soviet psychiatrists whom we have condemned for the unethical political abuse of psychiatry. If one has a dialogue with these Soviet forensic psychiatrists, one of the first points they make is that for them, the revolution is the greatest good for the greatest number. The greatest piece of social justice in the twentieth century is the greatest beneficence imaginable. It is when these psychiatrists act in the service of that beneficence that we believe their ethical compass as psychiatrists begins to wander. The scandals in medical research in this country demonstrate the same theme.[34] The advancement of science is a noble goal; you may prefer it to the revolution, or to the American system of justice, but when doctors give it greater weight than helping their patients or doing no harm they lose their ethical boundaries.

THE ADVERSARIAL STANDARD

It is sometimes said by forensic psychiatrists that all of the supposed ethical problems which have been rehearsed here do not exist because I have failed to recognize the avowedly adversarial nature of forensic testimony. These forensic psychiatrists would argue that they openly accept the fact that they have been selected in a biased fashion to be partisan expert witnesses. They have no ethical problems because they openly accept the responsibility of putting forward the best possible case for their side. Furthermore, they could argue that the ethics and value of such adversarial testimony is in fact as intelligible as it is for lawyers. But their assumption must be that this practice is ethical because, just as is the case with lawyers, it is understood by all of the participants in the system of Justice and no one is misled.

But does the jury clearly understand this partisan role of the forensic psychiatrist? After all, they watch as the forensic psychiatrist takes an oath to tell the truth, the whole truth, and not the partisan truth. The psychiatrist does not begin by revealing to the jury that he or she has been retained to make the best case possible. Rather, he or she is introduced to the jury with an impressive presentation of distinguished credentials to establish expertise, not partisanship or bias.

Nor does the judge instruct the jury that they should keep in mind, in weighing the expert testimony, that the forensic psychiatrists have an "ethical" responsibility to be biased. The jury is not told that even the most prestigious and convincing expert should be understood as having attempted to present the best case possible. Until there is this kind of candor in the courtroom, it will be impossible to sweep the ethical problems of psychiatry under the rug of intelligible adversarial ethics. And if the forensic psychiatrist is an explicit adversarial witness, think of how the intellectual problems will be solved! This may be an intelligible solution of the ethical boundaries, but it will certainly expose the limitations of our scientific and intellectual boundaries.

None of these are simple matters and I do not mean to suggest that they are or that I have any answers. What I have tried to do in this essay is to suggest that from the vantage point of the ivory tower, the intellectual and the ethical problems are inescapably linked.

Forensic psychiatry is caught on the horns of an ethical dilemma. It is a painful position to be in, but the greater danger is to think that one has found a more comfortable position: that one can simply adjust to the adversarial system or remain true to one's calling as a physician. The philosophers say life is a moral adventure; I would add that to choose a career in forensic psychiatry is to choose to increase the risks of that moral adventure. Those risks will become more obvious as we examine the testimony given in the Hinckley trial.

REFERENCES

1. Morse, Failed Explanations and Criminal Responsibility, *Virginia Law Review*, Vol. 68, pp. 971–1084 (1982).

2. *See, e.g., Bulletin of the American Academy of Psychiatry and the Law; Criminal Justice and Behavior; International Journal of Law and Psychiatry; International Journal of Offender Therapy and Comparative Criminology; Journal of Forensic Sciences; Journal of the Forensic Science Society; Journal of Psychiatry and Law; Law and Human Behavior; Law and Psychology Review; Mental Disability Law Reporter.*

3. American Psychiatric Association, *The Principles of Medical Ethics with Annotations Especially Applicable to Psychiatry*, Washington, D.C., 1981.

4. *Barefoot v. Estelle*, 103 S.Ct. 3383 (1983).

5. I. Kant, *Anthropology from a Pragmatic Point of View*, translated by V. L. Dowdell (Southern Illinois Univ. Press, 1978), p. 111.

6. *Ibid.*, p. 111.

7. Freud, Moral Responsibility for the Content of Dreams, cited in Katz, Goldstein and Dershowitz, *Psychoanalysis, Psychiatry and Law* (Free Press, 1967), p. 127.

8. H. Hartmann, *Psychoanalysis and Moral Values* (International Universities Press, 1960).

9. J. Goldstein, A. Freud, and A. Solnit, *Beyond the Best Interests of the Child* (Free Press, 1973) and *Before the Best Interests of the Child* (Free Press, 1980).

10. E. Furman, *A Child's Parent Dies* (Yale University Press, 1974).

11. Morse, *op. cit.*

12. S. Hook, ed., *Dimensions of Mind: A Symposium* (New York University Press, 1960).

13. *Matter of Torsney*, 412 N.Y.S.2d 914, *rev'd* 420 N.Y.S.2d 192, 394 N.E.2d 262.

14. M. S. Moore, Legal Conceptions of Mental Illness, in *Mental Illness: Law and Public Policy*, B. Brody and T. Englehardt, eds. (Kluwer Academic, 1980).

15. T. Kuhn, *The Structure of Scientific Revolutions*, ed. (University of Chicago Press, 1970), p. 2.

16. W. D. Hudson, ed., *The Is/Ought Question* (St. Martins Press, 1970).

17. Moore, Responsibility and the Unconscious, *Southern California Law Review*, Vol. 53, pp. 1563–1675 (1980).

18. N. Walker, *Crime and Insanity in England*, Vol. 1 (Edinburgh University Press, 1968), p. 82.

19. J. Ashbrook, The Insanity Defense, *Congressional Record*, Nov. 17, 1981, E 5365-6.

20. Kant, *op. cit.*, p. 111.

21. F. Redlich and J. Bingham, *The Inside Story: Psychiatry and Everyday Life* (Knopf, 1953).

22. M. Weber, Objectivity in Social Science and Social Policy, in *The Methodology of the Social Sciences*, translated by E. Shils and H. Finch (Free Press, 1949).

23. J. Rappeport, Ethics and Forensic Psychiatry, in *Psychiatric Ethics*, S. Bloch and P. Chodoff, eds. (Oxford University Press, 1981), p. 259.

24. *Ibid.*, p. 264.

25. J. Dedek, *Contemporary Medical Ethics* (Sheed and Ward, 1975), p. 6.

26. *But see* Rappeport, *op. cit.*, pp. 258–59. Rappeport believes it *is* possible to testify honestly and effectively. He argues that the limits of our knowledge will be made evident, so long as we do not try to confuse the issue or suggest that we have knowledge which we in fact lack.

27. S. Pollack, *Forensic Psychiatry in Criminal Law* (University of Southern California Press, 1974).

28. Bazelon, The Role of the Psychiatrist in the Criminal Justice System, *Bulletin of the American Academy of Psychiatry and Law*, Vol. 6, pp. 139–146 (1978).

29. Nor did the Court in *Barefoot* state that such testimony was unethical. Rather, it upheld the practice of allowing psychiatrists to respond to hypothetical questions about a person they had never examined.

30. *Estelle v. Smith*, 451 U.S. 454 (1981).

31. Oath or Affirmation Governing Principles, Form 161, Oath of Witness, 25 *Am. Jur. Pl. and Pr. Forms* (revised), pp. 356–357.

32. "The Unconscious of a Conservative: A Special Issue on the Mind of Barry Goldwater," *Fact Magazine*, Vol. 1, pp. 3–64, September-October 1964.

33. *Barefoot v. Estelle*, 103 S.Ct. 3383 (1983).

34. *See, e.g.,* discussion of cancer research in Jay Katz, *Experimentation with Human Beings: The Authority of the Investigator, Subject, Professions and State in the Human Experimentation Process* (Russell Sage, 1972).

IV

The Trial of John Hinckley

THE TRIAL OF JOHN HINCKLEY was a bleak experience for American psychiatry, and the verdict shook public confidence in the American criminal justice system. Criticism went in two directions: outrage against the law and outrage against psychiatry. Months before the assassination attempt, Hinckley had been arrested for attempting to carry guns onto an airplane. He had also been under private psychiatric care. But neither the law nor psychiatry had recognized that Hinckley was dangerous. There had been no protection for the public, and now there was to be no punishment for Hinckley. Indeed, given the judicial interpretation of the statutes governing the subsequent confinement of persons found not guilty by reason of insanity, there was a real possibility that Hinckley might regain his freedom.

There were many who thought the law was out of joint. Responding to public outrage, politicians talked about abolishing the insanity defense. Even before the trial began, Congressman Ashbrook of Ohio took aim at psychiatry. He described psychiatrists as "bogeymen" who know as much about the human mind as the butcher, the baker, and the candlestick maker.[1] It was time to get tough on crime and to throw the psychiatric pharisees out of the temple of law.

No informed and honest politician believes that abolition of the insanity defense is a way to get tough on crime. The crime rate in cities like New York staggers the imagination. One well-known statistical study showed that in 1940, a citizen of Manhattan had one chance in ten of being the victim of a serious crime in the course of a lifetime. By 1970 the risk had grown to only a little better than one chance in ten of *not* being a victim. Yet criminals are today less likely to be arrested, less likely to go to prison, and more apt to serve shorter sentences than they were in 1940.[2] The jails and prisons are filled beyond capacity; more and more violence is committed by juveniles, and no one seriously believes in rehabilitation.

These failures are starkly demonstrated by the statistics presented in the chapter on Psychiatry and Violence. There are currently 1,300,000 United States citizens who have been convicted of a crime and are on probation. Almost a quarter of a million Americans have served time in prison and are now out on parole. Over 400,000 people are incarcerated.[3] Thus, despite the statistical unlikelihood that a person who commits a criminal act will be arrested and convicted for that act,[4] nearly one out of every hundred Americans is a convicted criminal. These realities have little to do with psychiatry or the insanity defense. Abolishing the insanity defense will not make the large cities of America safer places in which to live. Psychiatry has every right to protest being made the scapegoat for the failures of the criminal justice system.

Many responsible politicians have recognized these bleak realities of the criminal justice system, and they acknowledge at least in private that the insanity defense is important only as a symbol. It has become a symbol of the impotence and unfairness of the criminal justice system. But it is only a symbol and not the reality.

At the same time, it is more difficult to keep these painful realities in public awareness than it is simply to blame psychiatry. And psychiatry is an easy target no matter how excellent the expert psychiatric witnesses may be—and they were impressive in the Hinckley trial. Consider the public's perception. They are shown again and again on television the horror of the assassination attempt. The violence could not be more real or terrifying. They want something done about it; if there is not retribution then at least the system of justice must condemn this violence. Instead, what the public is given is a confusing and conflicting set of arguments about legal insanity. In such a context, psychiatry will always be the loser even when the verdict is legally just, as I believe it was in the Hinckley case. By legally just, I mean that the verdict was fully compatible with the psychiatric testimony, the applicable legal test, and the burdens of proof.

CHANGING THE INSANITY DEFENSE

In hearings held immediately after the Hinckley verdict, Senator Specter of Pennsylvania accepted the possibility that the verdict was legally just, but he pointed out that this was because "the Congress had for two centuries allowed judges to formulate the insanity defense."[5] The judges had been too much influenced by the liberal academics who had, for example, formulated the American Law Institute's test, which judges had made into the law in most jurisdictions. He called on the elected members of Congress to assert control and promulgate a new test that would restrict the insanity defense and would exclude its use by defendants like Hinckley, who obviously *intended* to do violence when they committed violent acts.

This movement to restrict the insanity defense has swept the nation. New laws restricting the defense—and some calling for its abolition—have been introduced both in Congress and in state legislatures.

The American Psychiatric Association quickly reacted to this public and political outrage by proposing its own set of restrictions, which were received enthusiastically by the national media and soon adopted in their essence by the American Bar Association.[6] The APA proposal has also been well received in state and federal legislatures considering new legislation. The APA proposal involves retaining the insanity defense, but limiting it to those who have a serious mental illness such as psychosis. If this criterion of psychosis were to be implemented, some of the recent controversial insanity defense cases—involving such diagnoses as multiple personality, compulsive gambling, and combat stress syndrome—would not be possible. One judge has already taken a step in this direction. The court refused to allow a defendant charged with the interstate transportation of stolen goods to present psychiatric evidence of his "compulsive gambling disorder," holding that it was "questionable whether such a disorder . . . amounts to a mental disease as that concept has long been understood by the criminal law."[7] In addition to setting a higher threshold before the insanity defense could be asserted, the APA adopted only the cognitive prong of the two-pronged ALI test—"*a person is not responsible for criminal conduct if . . . he lacks substantial capacity either to appreciate the criminality [wrongfulness] of his conduct*"—and rejected the second prong—"*or to conform his conduct to the requirements of law.*"[8] It was the two-pronged ALI test that was applied to John Hinckley, and it has since become politically unpopular. The APA's spokesman, Dr. Loren

Roth, rejecting the ability-to-conform prong (also known as the volitional or "irresistible impulse" part of the test), commented in the APA position paper that "the line between an irresistible impulse and an impulse not resisted is probably no sharper than that between twilight and dusk."[9] In contrast, the APA believed that bright lines could be drawn about the presence or absence of a thought disorder, which would be relevant to the cognitive test of criminal responsibility. The APA presented their version of the cognitive test as a stricter standard and a more reliable one from a psychiatric perspective.

PSYCHIATRIC TESTIMONY IN THE COURTROOM

A basic theme of the APA's proposal was to get psychiatrists to practice psychiatry in the courtroom and not to try to practice law or morality. It was also hoped that if psychiatrists practiced psychiatry there might be less of a "battle of experts" and more of the diagnostic reliability that psychiatrists have achieved with the APA's official *Diagnostic and Statistical Manual of Mental Disorders,* Third Edition. DSM-III now specifies in great detail the symptoms and other criteria which must be present in order to make a particular diagnosis. Psychiatric diagnostic reliability, consistency between psychiatrists, has been dramatically improved through the use of the detailed criteria in DSM-III. Toward this end of psychiatrists practicing psychiatry, the APA would no longer allow psychiatric testimony about the ultimate legal question of criminal responsibility in cases in which they offer expert opinions.

But what exactly does this distinction mean? Every accepted legal test of insanity begins by asking whether "*by reason of* a mental disease (disorder) or defect *the person lacks*" whatever. If the APA proposal means that the psychiatrist is not to testify about anything in this sentence except "mental disease (disorder) or defect," then the proposal is radical indeed.

Recall that using the APA approach the jurors would first have to decide whether the defendant was psychotic based on the expert testimony. Then, if the psychiatrists did not offer their expert opinion about the effects of a psychosis, the jury, based on their own lay knowledge, would have to decide whether *by reason of* this psychosis the person "*lacked the substantial capacity to appreciate the wrongfulness. . . .* " The APA proposal, understood in this way, would seem to shift all of the theoretical problems outlined in the prior chapter from the psychiatrists to the jurors. The jurors would have to struggle with the question of what it means to say "*by reason of psychosis.*" They would have to solve the problems of free will versus determinism and the relationship between brain and mind and so forth. Perhaps it is a cynical view about jury deliberation, but it seems that under those circum-stances, everything would turn on the question, how psychotic was the defendant? And are not all the theoretical questions posed in the prior chapter buried under the concept of psychosis? And if, on the other hand, the psychiatrists do explain how psychosis affects the capacity to appreciate, what difference does it make whether they testify about the ul-timate legal question? The intellectual problems described in the last chapter are not located only in ultimate legal questions. If they are not bur-ied under the concepts of psychosis they certainly are to be found when the psychiatrist tries to explain how psychosis affects understanding.

Putting these more difficult theoretical questions to one side, let us consider what happened at the Hinckley trial. Would the APA proposal to have psychiatrists practice psychiatry rather than law or morality have produced less of a battle of experts? Would psychiatric testimony have been less controversial if the testimony had been confined to diagnostic criteria about thought disorder rather than volition? What are the implications of all this for American psychiatry? These questions will be discussed with reference to the trial transcript of the psychiatric testimony in the Hinckley trial.

Although all of the expert witnesses in the Hinckley trial have been identified in the media and some have appeared on national television, this chapter will focus on the substance of their ideas, rather than on the personalities involved. There will be controversy enough in the substance of their testimony. The psychiatrists will, therefore, be designated by impressionistic sobriquets—fanciful appellations. The trial record is, of course, a public document, and it has already been used as the basis of a fourteen million dollar malpractice suit, brought by three victims of Hinckley's bullets, against John Hinckley's psychiatrist, "Dr. Defendant." It is interesting to note that the lawsuit was brought not by a contingency fee lawyer, but by a public interest law firm concerned about the rights of victims. They have sued Hinckley himself for twenty-eight million dollars. Hinckley, unlike most criminal defendants, supposedly has "deep pockets," but this is unusual and even Hinckley's money is allegedly protected by some legal trust. As of this writing, the complaint against Hinckley's psychiatrist has been dismissed, but an appeal is expected.[10] It is the psychiatrist's malpractice insurance policy which has become the target of victims, as we shall see in a subsequent chapter.

NONPSYCHIATRIC CONSIDERATIONS

Before considering the psychiatric testimony, it is worth mentioning that we now know several things about the trial which may have influenced the result and which have nothing to do with psychiatric testimony. First, Hinckley—like Son of Sam, and like Mark David Chapman who killed John Lennon—preferred to plead guilty and plea bargain rather than to go to trial, but the prosecution refused. The prosecution's refusal to plea bargain seems to suggest that the prosecution was convinced that they could defeat an insanity plea. Second, Hinckley might possibly have been tried in the Criminal Court of the District of Columbia. Instead, he was tried in the Federal District Court, where the prosecution assumed the legal burden of proving Hinckley's sanity beyond a reasonable doubt. In the federal courts the prosecution assumes this burden of proof once a defendant successfully rebuts the presumption of legal sanity.[11] In contrast, in the District of Columbia Criminal Court, the burden would have been on Hinckley to prove his insanity by a preponderance of the evidence.[12] Not only, therefore, did the prosecution assume the burden of proof, they also had to prove sanity beyond a reasonable doubt. One simply has to credit the prosecution with being aware of the choice, and they chose the court which imposed the burden and the higher standard of proof on them.

Some reformers are now urging that the burden of proof be placed on the defendant in all courts. The APA has for good reasons left this technical legal question to the legislature. The American Bar Association has proposed that where the two-pronged ALI test including volition is maintained, the burden of proof should be on the defendant to prove his insanity by a preponderance of the evidence. Where the volitional test is not used, the ABA would support the requirement that the prosecution disprove the claim of insanity beyond a reasonable doubt.[13] Given this ABA recommendation made in response to the Hinckley verdict, it is worth considering whether Hinckley would have been found guilty using only the cognitive part of the ALI test but under the same burden of proof, that is, beyond a reasonable doubt.

Third, it has been said that the judge before whom the Hinckley case was tried was laboring under the impression that the jury would surely bring in a guilty verdict. Trial judges tend to have a vested interest in protecting their verdicts from being reversed by higher courts. This concern must have weighed heavily on a judge presiding at the trial of a man who attempted to kill the President. If such a judge thinks the jury will convict in any event, he or she may bend over backwards to avoid reversible error, and this effort may have the effect of favoring the defense, particularly in such matters as admitting evidence and in charging the jury. This is what the judge is said to have done in the Hinckley trial. Hinckley's lawyers do not agree with this hypothesis. The judge in their view was naturally concerned about reversible error in such an important trial, but their opinion is that this did not lead him to favor the defense.[14]

Fourth, the composition of a jury can be crucial in any trial—civil or criminal. Indeed, elaborate social science methods have been devised to assist counsel in selecting jury members.[15] The defense in the Hinckley trial was particularly concerned that their jury panel was predominantly black and poorly educated. They were concerned that jurors from such a background would be hostile to a wealthy defendant and also worried that they would be hostile towards complicated psychiatric testimony and psychiatric explanations and excuses for Hinckley's behavior. In fact, five of eleven black jurors in the case had had relatives hospitalized with serious mental illnesses, and therefore had first-hand experience with the reality of mental illness.

Finally, in addition to the young psychiatrist at the federal facility where Hinckley had been confined, the prosecution had retained three distinguished forensic psychiatrists to testify that Hinckley was not insane. After only one of them had testified, the prosecution decided not to call the others. Apparently, like the judge, the prosecution thought the case had been won. The judge, the prosecutor, the public, and most of the commentators expected a conviction, yet the jury's verdict was not guilty by reason of insanity. At any jury trial, the legal strategy and the performance of the attorneys is of great consequence. Surely the result in this trial had at least as much to do with the lawyers as with the psychiatrists.

PSYCHIATRIC TESTIMONY AT THE HINCKLEY TRIAL

The first psychiatrist to testify was Doctor Defendant; he was not sworn in as an expert witness. Rather, as John Hinckley's psychiatrist before the assassination attempt, his job was to try to explain his clinical judgment and a treatment that the whole world knew had failed. It is not an overstatement to suggest that Doctor Defendant was himself on trial, and the verdict in his case was guilty.

Reading the testimony one gets the impression that Doctor Defendant's approach had been directive, behavioral, reality, and family oriented rather than psychodynamic or psychoanalytic. Other treatment modalities included Valium and biofeedback to deal with anxiety and tension. Perhaps because the patient was being coerced into treatment by his parents, there seems never to have been real rapport. John Hinckley told Doctor Defendant almost nothing about his desperate and grandiose violent fantasy life or the actions he had taken and was taking in connection with those fantasies. Thus, Doctor Defendant's reality and family oriented treatment (in the 20/20 wisdom of hindsight) was out of touch with the fantasy and reality of John Hinckley.

Recently John Hinckley's parents appeared on national television and intimated that they believe their son had a schizophrenic disorder that Doctor Defendant had failed to diagnose. And psychiatrists at the Hinckley trial have said that Doctor Defendant's approach and treat-ment were wrong, that his prescription of biofeedback and Valium were contraindicated, and that he should have recognized the lack of rapport as symptomatic of Hinckley's condition. It is apparent how the expert testimony on behalf of Hinckley would seem to provide most of the legal research on the standard of care necessary for a malpractice suit. If the malpractice case against Doctor Defendant is reinstated on appeal, psychiatry once again will be tried in the media and no doubt will again be found lacking, whatever the verdict.

As the trial transcript reveals, Doctor Defendant left the stand desperately wanting to say something more about his former patient which he thought would help the court in its deliberations, but since he had not been sworn in as an expert witness he was forbidden to do so by the judge.

Eventually other psychiatrists would be presented as expert wit-nesses, and the jury would hear all of their diagnostic jargon. The DSM-III diagnoses offered by the three psychiatrists for the defense included schizophrenia, schizotypal personality disorder with psychosis, and borderline and paranoid personality disorder with psychosis. A diagno-sis of major depressive episode was considered also tenable, but it was suggested that this was secondary to the schizophrenic disorder.[16]

The defense psychiatrists also mentioned as appropriate diagnoses, even though not included in DSM-III, schizophrenic spectrum disor-der, process schizophrenia, simple schizophrenia, pseudoneurotic schizophrenia, and ambulatory schizophrenia. The psychiatrists for the prosecution confined themselves to the DSM-III classification, but they diagnosed narcissistic personality disorder, schizoid personality disorder, mixed personality disorder with borderline and passive/aggressive fea-tures, and dysthymic disorder. One can only sympathize with the jurors.

They would have needed to be sequestered for a week with Robert Spitzer (Chairman of the APA's DSM-III task force) just to digest the nosological jargon.

One bill proposed to Congress and advocated by a psychiatrist would not only bar psychiatrists from expressing their opinion about the ultimate legal question of insanity, it would also ban the psychiatrist from offering a diagnosis.[17] This solution might be a relief to the judge and jury, but it would not have eliminated much of the confusion and controversy in the Hinckley trial. In fact, DSM-III played a rather interesting and important role in the testimony. The core of the diagnostic dispute comes down to whether Hinckley had a thought disorder, a perfect test for the APA's new proposal. All of the defense psychiatrists said he did. But the prosecution found no thought disorder and they rejected even those DSM-III personality disorders which are most suggestive of thought disorder—schizotypal and paranoid personality. Thus, to the extent that the experts practiced psychiatry in accordance with the APA proposal, there was profound disagreement about one of the most basic aspects of a psychiatric evaluation, the presence or absence of a thought disorder. Given this kind of disagreement, it seems quite unlikely that removing diagnoses from psychiatric testimony would make the jury's job easier. Psychiatrists can inject just as much jargon without mentioning diagnosis. And in the Hinckley trial, the diagnostic jargon of DSM-III put certain contraints on the testimony. The specification of diagnoses in DSM-III allowed lawyers during the Hinckley trial to cross-examine more effectively, that is, to ask why, given certain symptoms, a particular diagnosis was not made.

The first psychiatrist for the defense, Doctor Researcher, gave a detailed anamnesis. He described a pattern of growing social isolation, failure, unhappiness, and suicidal ideation.[18] Against this background, Hinckley created a fantasy world of unrealistic, bizarre, and grandiose expectation. He began to have ideas of reference and magical thinking. He travelled all over the country: to Hollywood to become a song writer,[19] to Yale to rescue Jodie Foster,[20] to Memphis to assassinate President Carter.[21] Having failed at everything, he went home and made a suicide attempt.[22] This is what led to his therapy with Doctor Defendant. During therapy Hinckley's condition further deteriorated. Doctor Defendant apparently was concerned that Hinckley's parents were reinforcing dependency and failure. Based on this conception, he advised the family not to take Hinckley back into their home after another cross-country excursion that led to failure. The father took this advice and refused to be supportive. Hinckley left Colorado. He alternated between suicidal thoughts and grandiose identification with the hero of the movie "Taxi Driver," Travis Bickle, and with John Lennon and with his assassin.[23] He ended up in Washington where he tried to assassinate President Reagan—a grandiose historic deed that would make him famous and unite him perhaps in death with the delusional love object, Jodie Foster.[24]

For those of us who have tried to understand the subjective, psychodynamic experience of schizophrenia, Doctor Researcher's testimony was compelling. Doctor Researcher was convinced that Hinckley demonstrated features that are pathognomonic of schizophrenia.[25] He described Hinckley's condition as process schizophrenia and concluded that Hinckley could neither appreciate the wrongfulness of his actions nor conform.

Doctor Biological Psychiatry, the second witness for the defense, saw Hinckley's condition as schizophrenia spectrum disorder.[26] Hinckley had a "very diseased or sick mind."[27] He described DSM-III as the "statute law of psychiatry,"[28] a "noble" but apparently, in his view, not entirely successful attempt to divide up the schizophrenia spectrum disorder. He described Hinckley as "the man with schizophrenia who had all the negative symptoms, but he didn't have the florid positive symptoms."[29] By negative symptoms he meant Eugen Bleuler's four A's: loose associations, autism, pathological ambivalence, and disorder of affect. "This is what I mean by schizophrenia: there are four abnormalities."[30] He emphasized and pushed the diagnosis of simple schizophrenia as appropriate to describe such a patient. Simple schizophrenia has been eliminated from DSM-III.

One of the controversial points in Doctor Biological Psychiatry's testimony was his attempt to introduce results of computerized axial tomography (CAT-scan) as evidence of abnormality in Hinckley's brain. The CAT-scan demonstrated widened sulci [the shallow furrows on the surface of the brain], but not enlarged ventricles.[31] The admissibility of the CAT-scan created a legal controversy of its own. Doctor Biological Psychiatry testified that he ordered CAT-scans for 70 percent of his patients and that Hinckley's CAT-scan "increases the possibility of the diagnosis being schizophrenic and decreases the possibility of personality disorder."[32] He suggested that the "scientific community accepts" the connection between widened sulci and schizophrenia.[33] The prosecution psychiatrists, although acknowledging the possible importance of CAT-scan research, compared it to other false leads in the study of schizophrenia, like the "pink spot" [once thought to demonstrate the presence of a particular substance in the blood][34] or the relation between the double Y chromosome and violence.[35] One prosecution psychiatrist testified that Blue Cross/Blue Shield would not pay for a CAT-scan to establish a diagnosis of schizophrenia, in order to demonstrate that the test was not generally accepted for the diagnostic purposes Doctor Biological Psychiatry claimed for it.[36]

Eventually the CAT-scan was declared admissible—perhaps because the judge was bending over backwards to be fair to the defendant. At least one juror said that it made no impression on him. However, Doctor Biological Psychiatry did not rely on CAT-scan evidence alone. John Hinckley was a would-be songwriter, poet, story writer, and diarist. The defense psychiatrists, particularly Doctor Biological Psychiatry, often referred to this material as demonstrating and confirming their clinical findings of thought disorder.

Doctor Clinician, the final psychiatric witness for the defense, reviewed and summed up the defense's case by emphasizing eight points in Hinckley's history and mental status: (1) progressive social isolation, (2) identity disturbance, (3) pathological absorption in fantasy, (4) self-damaging impulsivity, (5) depression with somatic symptoms, (6) peculiar mental experiences including ideas of reference and a great deal of magical thinking, (7) difficulties with anger and ambivalence, and (8) inhibition of normal heterosexual behavior. He saw Hinckley as a schizotypal personality who had become psychotic before he shot the President. He, like Doctor Biological Psychiatry, would have diagnosed Hinckley as a simple schizophrenic under DSM-II (the previous edition of DSM-III).

Doctor Forensics, the first prosecution psychiatrist, set about recasting the history. He brought out four main themes: advantages, entitlement, premeditation, and manipulation. In place of psychological hardship and painful isolation, he saw advantages, luxurious surroundings, and a spoiled rich kid. Where the defense psychiatrists saw failure and frustration, he saw entitlement and easy living. Where they saw a suicide attempt he saw a suicidal gesture. Where they saw acting out of a delusional fantasy, he saw premeditation. Finally, where they saw isolation and inability to deal with others, he saw deception, dishonesty, and clever manipulation to get what Hinckley wanted.

He suggested that Hinckley had manipulated and deceived the defense psychiatrists. And he was, in fact, able to identify a number of inconsistencies between the facts and their impressions. For example, Hinckley had three kinds of bullets. He selected from this arsenal six exploding devastator bullets. This selection, whether conscious or unconscious, apparently was an objective fact.[37] The defense psychiatrists had accepted Hinckley's statement that he had grabbed bullets at random. They had relied on this statement for their clinical impression that he had been in a psychotic state and that there had been no premeditation. Doctor Forensics criticized the use of poetry for diagnos-ing thought disorder. He suggested that on that basis our mental hospitals would contain all of our greatest poets.[38] It is worth mention-ing that the jury during their deliberations asked for a dictionary. They wanted to see whether poetry was defined as fiction or nonfiction. It is not clear what turned on that distinction but it suggests that the psychiatric disagreement about the significance of Hinckley's poetry was of concern to the jury.

Doctor Forensics carefully applied the "statute law" of DSM-III and concluded that Hinckley could be diagnosed in at least four personality disorder categories,[39] but he was not psychotic and he was certainly responsible for his actions.[40] DSM-III requires the psychiatrist to demonstrate the presence of several diagnostic criteria as manifest by at least a certain number of symptoms. The key to the prosecution's disagreement with the defense's DSM-III diagnoses was their conflict-ing judgment about whether a given mental trait or behavior pattern was present and, if so, whether or not it amounted to a symptom. Some examples are mentioned below.

Doctor Corrections, another psychiatrist for the prosecution, had been the first to evaluate Hinckley after his arrest and confinement in the federal facility at Butner. Her evaluation therefore must be given special weight. She detected no symptoms of schizophrenia as they are set out in DSM-III and the diagnostic decision tree presented there. Nor had she found magical thinking, illusions, ideas of reference, or a family history of schizophrenia. She therefore eliminated a diagnosis of schizotypal disorder and paranoid personality disorder, as had Doctor Forensics. She saw Hinckley's self-importance, manipulation, and egocentricity as all compatible with a narcissistic personality disorder.[41] She emphasized his lying, envy, irresponsible behavior, depression, and blaming others as characteristic of traits commonly seen in people with narcissistic personality disorder.

ACCOUNTING FOR THE CONFLICTING TESTIMONY

How are we to understand these radical discrepancies between the defense and prosecution psychiatrists' diagnoses? The defense experts seem to have adopted the traditional nonconfrontational interviewing style with Hinckley that most of us would use when dealing with ordinary patients. They believed the patient, and they looked for psychopathology the way we psychiatrists usually do. Perhaps they were conned by Hinckley. The prosecution experts, in contrast, challenged Hinckley's assertions, confronted contradictions, and checked the objective evidence against his statements. They assumed he might be trying to con them. Perhaps they made him defensive. They combined ordinary psychiatric skills and police investigation techniques. There must have been radical differences in the emotional climate of the interviews. The different emotional climates may well have influenced the perceptions of pathology. For example, where the defense saw flattened and inappropriate affect, the prosecution saw a demanding manipulative person who was aware of what was going on, wanted special treatment, and had only a little blunting of affect.

In this connection, the defense psychiatrist's testimony, whether correct and accurate or not, was not unlike what one expects to hear from a psychiatrist presenting a patient at a staff conference. The prosecution psychiatrists, on the other hand, seemed to reveal a kind of animus against Hinckley. Perhaps this was a result of their adversarial role. But it may be that when we conclude that someone is criminally responsible, we are also apt to become convinced that the person is hateful and contemptible. But if the prosecution psychiatrists had a certain animus, it must also be said that their picture of Hinckley may have been closer to the image he tried to portray. He had not wanted to plead insanity and there are other reasons to conclude that he wanted to seem calculating, manipulative, and inscrutable. Ironically, he seems to have had a need to appear in control of himself.

Of great interest was the weight and interpretation given to the same material by the two sides. Hinckley allegedly saw the movie "Taxi Driver" some fifteen times. He identified with and dressed like the protagonist, Travis Bickle, he memorized the music, perhaps he lived out the plot. Are these behaviors evidence of psychotic identification problems (as the defense psychiatrists argued) or do they amount to something much less (as the prosecution psychiatrists said)? Was his obsession with Jodie Foster a delusion, or was it merely unrealistic and inappropriate? When does a fantasy become a fixed idea? When does a fixed idea become a delusion?

Consider the differing interpretations given to more trivial facts. Hinckley reported that President Reagan was in the Hilton Hotel only about twenty minutes, when in fact he was there for almost forty-five minutes. The prosecution psychiatrist cited this as an example of his untrustworthiness as an informant. The defense gave this as an example of how the sense of time is distorted in psychotic panic. Hinckley bought the same kind of gun that had been used to kill John Lennon. The defense assumed that this was further evidence of his pathological identification. The prosecution said that he must have learned from media reports that the gun was small, flat, and unusually concealable.

And of course the psychiatrists were encouraged in many ways by the lawyers' questions to discredit more directly each other's testimony. Doctor Forensics criticized the defense psychiatrists for failing to interview witnesses who could have described Hinckley's demeanor at the time of the shooting, which he claimed was relevant to the evaluation of Hinckley's mental status at that time. Doctor Biological Psychiatry confessed that he was horrified at such supposedly standard forensic practices. "For state of mind evidence," such "casual observations are a very poor source, indeed a treacherous source of information."[42] Doctor Researcher described Hinckley as a straightforward informant. Doctor Corrections suggested that dishonesty was a basic feature of Hinckley's personality.

None of this conflicting testimony, which was the result of psychiatrists doing psychiatry in the courtroom, would have been eliminated by the APA's new restrictive test. Nor would it be eliminated by barring psychiatric diagnosis. The only way to eliminate such conflicts would be to eliminate psychiatric testimony.

Whatever their differing interpretations, the most distressing impression, reading the trial transcript, is created by the apparent certainty and conviction with which the experts expressed their psychiatric opinions, and the doggedness with which all but one of them maintained their certainty in the face of cross examination. The diagnosis of simple schizophrenia and Bleuler's four A's were presented by defense psychiatrists as the bedrock certainty of scientific psychiatry, despite the fact that during the past two decades serious questions have been raised about the validity of the diagnosis of simple schizophrenia and Bleuler's distinction between fundamental and accessory symptoms.[43] Despite these excesses, it would be impossible to say that these psychiatrists did not live up to the standards described in the previous chapter: the good clinical practice standard, the scientific standard, and the truth and honesty standard. As the Hinckley testimony reveals, these standards simply do not work if working means they would prevent psychiatrists from testifying in diametric opposition to each other. The only standard which accounts for this conflicting testimony is the adversarial standard, making the best case for your side. Let us now consider this conflicting testimony in light of the APA proposal's other requirements.

THE APA TEST IN LIGHT OF THE HINCKLEY TESTIMONY

Despite the endless attempts of law to define precise tests of criminal responsibility, the ordinary psychiatrist typically asks: Is the person psychotic? If the diagnosis is psychosis, particularly schizophrenia, the person is insane. If a personality disorder is diagnosed, the person is sane. The new APA proposal has gone back to that time-honored clinical distinction, noting that we now have 80 percent reliability as to the DSM-III diagnosis of psychosis. But this new threshold question would have had no impact on the Hinckley testimony since the defense diagnosed schizophrenia and the prosecution diagnosed personality disorder. Hinckley apparently fell into the 20 percent nonreliability category. We should not be surprised by that. Rather, we should expect that in most cases where the prosecution would want to contest an insanity defense, the defendant will not be obviously psychotic. The obviously psychotic defendant can be readily identified even by a prosecutor. Thus it may be that contested cases raising the insanity defense will be those about which we can expect diagnostic disagreement by psychiatrists. And as the Hinckley trial suggests, expert witnesses do not feel bound by the DSM-III diagnostic categories which have produced the 80 percent reliability.

The next part of the APA proposal involves going back to an essentially cognitive test—again in part because psychiatric testimony relevant to cognitive matters such as appreciation and understanding "is more reliable, and has a stronger scientific base"[44] than testimony relevant to volition. Here again the hopes of the APA proposal fail. The defense found ample evidence of thought disorder, including ideas of reference, magical thinking, bizarre ideas, and a break with reality. The prosecution found none of this. Thus testimony limited to the cognitive issue did not prove reliable in the courtroom.

This lack of reliability in diagnosing thought disorder also raises questions about the ABA's decision that where the restrictive cognitive test is adopted, the burden of proving beyond a reasonable doubt that the defendant is not insane should remain with the prosecution. Presumably this decision was made on the premise that this burden of proof would be lightened by the narrower test, which would draw brighter lines. The transcript of the trial suggests that this did not happen in the Hinckley case. Given the psychiatric testimony, there would have been reasonable doubt about Hinckley's insanity even as to the narrower cognitive test. If the ABA's decision was made with the Hinckley verdict in mind and intended to produce a different result in similar cases, it fails based on this analysis.

The discrepancies in the psychiatric testimony would be much easier to understand if the defense and prosecution had agreed that there was a thought disorder but disagreed about its extent—for example, whether it was sufficient to be diagnosed psychosis, and whether it was sufficient to negate criminal responsibility. Such agreement would have placed Hinckley in the problem area of psychiatry's familiar nosological disputes. Thus, if both sides had agreed that he was a schizotypal personality or a paranoid personality and the defense said he had gone over into psychosis while the prosecution insisted he had not, every clinician would have understood the problem. How much thought disorder makes a psychosis? But here the prosecution specifically rejected the diagnoses of schizotypal personality and paranoid personality, the character disorders which suggest a thought disorder. This makes the discrepancies harder to understand and harder to explain to the cynics who believe psychiatrists can be hired to say anything.

A SUGGESTED DIAGNOSIS FOR JOHN HINCKLEY

Based on my own reading of the testimony of all the psychiatrists, I believe that before DSM-III, I would have diagnosed John Hinckley as a case of erotomania, and Freud's classic paper written in 1911[45] would have helped me to clarify Hinckley's psychopathology. Most clinicians have seen patients with delusions of love—a condition that is not that uncommon. There is even a French name for such delusions—Clerambault's syndrome. In fact, the man who killed Tatiana Tarasoff and created the *Tarasoff* case[46] seems to have had the same kind of pathology as John Hinckley. But erotomania per se no longer appears in DSM-III, and one could debate whether it is or is not a psychosis. It is my own clinical and theoretical opinion that a delusion of love may protect the person against ego decompensation into florid psychosis, and this may have been the case with Hinckley. His pathological attachment to Jodie Foster is in my view crucial not only to his diagnosis but also to his prognosis. It is interesting, however, that delusions of love seem to have disappeared from DSM-III. Such delusions do not make up a separate diagnosis and are not listed as a specific symptom in any of the diagnostic categories of the paranoid spectrum. Perhaps the Hinckley case may also lead us to reconsider this gap in DSM-III.

EVALUATING THE PSYCHIATRIC DIAGNOSES

The defense psychiatrists themselves had trouble finding a place for Hinckley in DSM-III. Whether they were oriented psychoanalytically or biologically, their theoretical understanding of the underlying disorder caused them to fight the atheoretical diagnostic categories of DSM-III. The defense's experts all had a more powerful commitment to their theory (biological, psychodynamic, or biopsychosocial) of Hinckley's psychiatric condition than they did to the diagnostic nomenclature in DSM-III. If they had been forbidden to use diagnoses (as already noted, some favor legislation that forbids diagnoses), they would have been released from a constraint against which they struggled. On the other hand, the prosecution witnesses seemed to have no theory about Hinckley's disorder and no real explanation of his actions except that he was a bad narcissistic person. Rather, they carefully and conscientiously applied DSM-III.

In evaluating these conclusions about the psychiatric testimony, several things should be kept in mind. First, the preparation and the quality of the psychiatric testimony in the Hinckley case was far superior to what one usually finds. Second, these experts appear to have genuinely and honestly come to their various conclusions. The Hinckley testimony is not an example of what happens when lawyers buy psychiatric experts for a price. The testimony may have been rehearsed, the experts may have been carefully sorted and selected by the lawyers, but these experts believed what they said. If Hinckley did not fall readily into any DSM-III category, if his disorder is in the gray area between psychosis and personality disorder, then we can see that there was room for honest disagreement.

Third, this presentation of the psychiatric testimony is taken from hundreds of pages of transcript. Everyone is therefore quoted out of context with an eye to emphasizing areas of disagreement. If there was something flawed about the psychiatric testimony, it is in the sense one gets of the psychiatrists getting caught up in and succumbing to the adversarial process. There is a kind of overstatement in their testimony as though they had taken on the responsibility of convincing the jury and outwitting the opposition. Clinical working hypotheses became scientific truths. Clinical possibilities became certainties. And as these truths and certainties from one side meet contradictory truths and certainties from the other side, one has the feeling that psychiatry's credibility hangs in the balance.

Whatever their own standards may have been, the psychiatrists' testimony reads as though the psychiatrists were following the adversary standard of lawyers—they were putting forward the best possible case for their side. But as was noted in the earlier chapter, they were not presented to the jury as advocates; they were sworn in as experts.

SOME TENTATIVE CONCLUSIONS

The jury reached a just decision in the Hinckley case if justice means a decision that adheres to existing law. There is no question that Hinckley had a serious mental disorder. He may not have been psychotic. But even the prosecution psychiatrists diagnosed four different kinds of DSM-III personality disorders, and there was certainly very good reason for the jurors to believe that Hinckley could have been psychotic, that he could have had a thought disorder, and that he could have lacked the substantial capacity to appreciate wrongfulness and to conform his behavior. The psychiatric testimony leaves one in doubt on these matters, but the burden was on the prosecution to remove that doubt. Under existing law the Hinckley verdict was a just result, and psychiatry has no reason to go on apologizing for that result.

The APA's new restrictive test would have made little difference in either the testimony or the verdict. It was the APA's intention to acknowledge that the ultimate legal question of insanity was of a kind which psychiatric expertise alone could not decide. The basic goal of the APA's proposal was to try to limit psychiatrists to what they do best: evaluating the mental status and condition of the defendant psychiatrically and medically.

The APA hoped that psychiatric testimony limited to what psychiatrists do best would be more exact, more reliable, and less controversial. The Hinckley transcript dashes those hopes. Most of the testimony was devoted to just those considerations, and yet the experts disagreed on every significant aspect of clinical evaluation: history, symptoms, mental status, and reliability of the informant.

The APA's narrowing of the insanity defense to the cognitive test would also have failed because the experts disagreed about whether

Hinckley had a thought disorder. Cognitive evaluation did not prove more reliable. There is the further, interesting issue of psychiatric testimony on ultimate legal questions. Until recently, courts allowed psychiatric testimony going to ultimate legal questions. In this respect, forensic psychiatry was antithetical to testimony in civil cases, in which witnesses traditionally have been barred from testifying about ultimate legal conclusions. However, the Federal Rules of Evidence, which govern practice in federal courts, have relaxed this long-standing barrier, allowing otherwise admissible opinion testimony that embraces an ultimate legal issue.[47] Recently, a federal judge seems to have accepted the APA's recommendation to exclude testimony regarding ultimate legal conclusions. "The psychiatrist is not called to offer his opinion as to the defendant's guilt, to characterize (in a usurpation of the jury's function) that state of mind as beyond lay comprehension, or to suggest that the defendant lacked control over his actions."[48] The ABA's Criminal Justice Mental Health Standards also follows this approach.[49] This, as was noted earlier, does not recognize that the insurmountable theoretical problems are not confined to the ultimate legal questions.

Everything the APA has proposed in response to the Hinckley verdict is thoughtful and sensible, and yet I believe it would have made no difference in the outcome of the Hinckley trial.

Changing the insanity defense is like chipping away at the tip of the iceberg. The rest of the iceberg consists of the deeper, more basic theoretical problems alluded to in the prior chapter. An exchange between defense and prosecution psychiatrists will illustrate one aspect of these deeper and more basic theoretical problems. Doctor Biological Psychiatry said that the Valium Hinckley took may well have produced "paradoxical rage," thus causing him to be unable to control himself. Doctor Corrections said it was "appropriate" for Hinckley to take Valium if he was anxious about assassinating the President. Put aside the fact that these are both conjectures. They are conjectures which are part of two quite different kinds of discourse.

The theory of paradoxical rage is part of a discourse about organisms with brains, enzymes, and physical chemical reactions. The theory of appropriate behavior is part of a discourse about persons with minds, intentions, and motivated actions. In the discourse about organisms, the self disappears and paradoxical rage is *caused* by the chemical release of the inhibitory neural system. In the discourse about persons, the self is the agent who chooses, who intends, and who assumes a firing position and pulls the trigger. Morality does not enter the discourse of organisms because free will and choice are not part of that language. To say that a *person* had a paradoxical rage reaction is to confuse the two discourses. The correct statement is that the organism was subject to a paradoxical rage reaction. (Even then the word rage is suspect.)

Psychiatry has not yet found a unified discourse about organisms and persons. That is the giant iceberg against which the insanity defense inevitably is wrecked. Neither psychiatry nor law nor moral philosophy has found a sure way past this barrier. It does no good to pre-tend the barrier does not exist or to ask the jury to deal with it. These are not questions for which common sense has an answer.

The insanity defense has been a symbol of the impotence and unfairness of the criminal justice system, but the insanity defense is also a symbol of the relationship between law and psychiatry. There was a time when psychiatrists were the ones urging an expanded insanity defense. There was a time when courts were urging us to tell them what to do. It seemed then that Freud's followers had gotten past the barrier. The best scholarly book on the insanity defense of that era, written by Abraham Goldstein,[50] looked to ego-psychology and the volitional half of the ALI test as the path of progress. The APA's return to the cognitive half of the test signals the end of that false hope and the beginning of a new one.

Psychiatry is held hostage by the psychiatrists who testify in courts whatever their standards and whatever the test of insanity may be. They undertake an enterprise which has hazards for us all. The reputation and credibility of our profession is in their hands. And if I am correct about the iceberg, they know not what they are doing.

REFERENCES

1. 127 *Congressional Record* E5365 (daily ed. Nov. 17, 1981) (Statement on Insanity Defense by J. Ashbrook).

2. S. Shinnar and R. Shinnar, The Effects of the Criminal Justice System on the Control of Crime: A Quantitative Approach, *Law and Society Review*, Vol. 9, p. 581, 1975.

3. *See, e.g.,* U.S. Department of Justice, *Governmental Responses to Crime; Vol. II, Crime and Governmental Responses in American Cities* (Government Printing Office, 1982).

4. Contrast conviction statistics with the FBI's Index of Crime, *Law Enforcement Bulletin*, No. B1, pp. 15–18, October 1903.

5. *Insanity Defense in Federal Courts, Hearings before the House Judiciary Committee, Subcommittee on Criminal Justice,* 97th Cong., 2d Sess. 2 (testimony of Senator Specter).

6. American Psychiatric Association, *Statement on the Insanity Defense,* December 1982. American Bar Association, *Criminal Justice Mental Health Standards* (First Tentative Draft), July 1983.

7. *See, United States v. Torniero,* 570 F. Supp. 721 (D. Conn. 1983), memorandum and order.

8. Model Penal Code, §4.01(1).

9. American Psychiatric Association, *Op. Cit.* note 6.

10. *Brady v. Hopper,* No. 83-JM-451 (D. Colo. 1983).

11. *Davis v. United States,* 160 U.S. 469 (1895), *Lynch v. Overholser,* 369 U.S. 705 (1962).

12. *See ABA Standards, Op. Cit.,* note 6 at sections 7.292–7.295.

13. *Ibid.*

14. Personal Communication.

15. *See, generally* N. L. Kerr and R. M. Bray, eds., *The Psychology of the Courtroom* (Academic Press, 1982). *See also, Jurimetrics Journal,* Vol. 23, pp. 321–324 (Spring, 1983).

16. p. 3803, trial transcript.

17. Glen Miller, personal communication.

18. pp. 3097–3119, trial transcript.

19. p. 3115, trial transcript.

20. pp. 3171–3174, trial transcript.

21. pp. 3174–3177, trial transcript.

22. p. 3184, trial transcript.

23. p. 3204, trial transcript.

24. pp. 3273, 3275, trial transcript.

25. pp. 3301–3304, trial transcript.

26. p. 3803, trial transcript.

27. p. 3835, trial transcript.

28. p. 3810, trial transcript.

29. pp. 3803, 3813, trial transcript.

30. p. 3805, trial transcript.

31. p. 5645, trial transcript.

32. pp. 3962–3963, trial transcript.

33. pp. 5389–5390, trial transcript.

34. pp. 5452–5454, trial transcript.

35. pp. 5467–5468, trial transcript.

36. p. 5470, trial transcript.

37. *See, e.g.*, p. 6450, trial transcript.

38. p. 7032, trial transcript.

39. pp. 7129–7131, 7225, trial transcript.

40. p. 7260, trial transcript.

41. p. 7537, trial transcript.

42. p. 4082, trial transcript.

43. A. Stone, R. Hopkins, et al., *Simple Schizophrenia—Syndrome or Shibboleth*, American Journal of Psychiatatry, Vol. 125, pp. 305–312 (1968).

44. APA Statement, *Op. Cit.* note 6.

45. J. Strachey, ed., On the Mechanism of Paranoia, *The Standard Edition of the Complete Psychological Works of Sigmund Freud* (The Hogarth Press, 1958).

46. *See, People v. Poddar*, 10 Cal.3d 750, 518 P.2d 342 (1974).

47. *See*, Advisory Committee Notes to Rule 704, Federal Rules of Evidence.

48. *See, e.g., U.S. v. Torneiro, op. cit.*, pp. 23–24.

49. ABA Standards, *Op. Cit.* note 6.

50. A. S. Goldstein, *The Insanity Defense* (Yale University Press, 1967).

V

Psychiatry and the Supreme Court

I N A LETTER TO HIS FATHER, Franz Kafka described his brief stay in law school as chewing on sawdust that had already been chewed on by hundreds of mouths before his. I am sure that any detailed attempt at describing how the Supreme Court has applied the Constitution to psychiatry would leave most readers picking sawdust out of their teeth.

Kafka has another, more intriguing vision of the law, which can be found in his great novel, *The Trial*. In it he tells of the peasant who seeks entrance to the law. The door to the law is open, but it is guarded by a great soldier. The peasant cajoles, begs, and bribes the guard to give him entry to the law. The guard refuses, and warns the peasant that this is only the first of many doors, each with more fearsome guards. Finally, after years of vain effort, the peasant, who has gotten to know every louse in the guard's fur coat, is near death. The guardian of the law is, of course, eternal, and quite unchanged by the passage of time.

As the moment of the peasant's death approaches, his sight begins to dim and in this darkness he sees a strange and wonderful light coming from the door of the law. But now a disturbing thought enters his mind. With his last strength, he beckons to the guard and asks, "Everyone strives to attain the law, how does it come about that in all these years, no one has come to this door seeking admittance but me?"

The guard, realizing that the peasant is dying, bends down to him, and shouts in his ear, "No one but you could gain admittance through this door, since this door was intended only for you. I am now going to shut it."

There have been days in my career when I have felt like Kafka's peasant at the first door of the law. Having listened to the learned faculty of the Harvard Law School for fifteen years, I know there are many, many doors and I have surely become familiar with the lawyers' fur coats. In this chapter, in the spirit of Kafka's peasant, I will explore some of the strange light I have seen coming from my own special door.

THE FIRST ILLUMINATION: LAW AS POLICY AND POLITICS

Justice Potter Stewart, in one of the cases I shall discuss, was quite candid about one of the central mysteries of the courts' law and psychiatry decisions. He wrote:

> Issues concerning mental illness are among the most difficult the courts have to face involving as they often do serious problems of policy disguised as questions of constitutional law.[1]

Thus, at least one member of the court recognized that dealing with the difficult problems of the mentally ill is not just a matter of determining Fourteenth Amendment requirements. This is an important and welcome revelation. Psychiatrists should not be intimidated by lawyers who dogmatically insist that the Constitution requires "X"!

I learned this early in my own career in law and psychiatry, when I found myself on the other side from the American Civil Liberties Union, in a case called Doe v. Roe.[2] The ACLU was assisting a New York psychiatrist who was attempting to publish a book-length case history of a patient's psychoanalysis, against the patient's wishes. The book contained the most intimate details and many stigmatizing interpretations of the patient's problems and personality. Through these descriptions, the patient was unnecessarily identifiable to her friends. The irony of this litigation was that with a few hours of careful editing the patient's identity could have been protected.

I had rallied both the American Psychiatric Association and the American Psychoanalytic Association to come in on the side of the patient and against the doctor. Marvin Karpatkin, then the lawyer for the ACLU, called me up to attempt to change my mind. Uttering all the high-sounding rhetoric of the First Amendment and prior restraint of free speech, Mr. Karpatkin, a forceful advocate, made me feel that I was either an enemy of civil liberties or an idiot peasant at the first door of the law.

I am a stubborn man, however, and I stuck to my moral intuition that what the doctor had done was stupid and wrong, and that no constitutional argument would make it right in this or in other cases that might follow from Karpatkin's reading of the Constitution. (It should be noted that at least a few psychiatrists in California had declared themselves ready to go to jail rather than reveal their patients' confidential communications. And there were lawyers who argued that such confidential communications were protected by the Constitution.) I am happy to say that with our help the patient prevailed and the First Amendment has survived without the sacrifice of the patient's privacy.

This anecdote drives home a more general point about applying the Constitution to the reform of psychiatry. In the leading Supreme Court law and psychiatry cases, the constitutional arguments frequently function merely as transparent window dressing for the Justices' own values, moral intuitions, and personal opinions. I do not deny that important rights are at issue, nor do I mean to suggest that the Constitution is irrelevant to psychiatry. But I am saying that in most of the law and psychiatry cases, Justice Stewart is correct; the Supreme Court is not applying the Constitution, it is struggling to resolve difficult questions of policy in an area that it knows little about. And what Justice Stewart did not say is that policy is influenced by politics even in the Supreme Court. I am describing the perspective from my particular door, but let me say that some of my colleagues at Harvard Law School who presumably have penetrated many doors of the law would claim that all Supreme Court decisions, in every field, involve questions of policy and politics disguised as narrow questions of constitutional law.

In this chapter I will be developing the point that the Supreme Court's dealings with psychiatry can be understood as involving three basic policy questions. First is what my late friend Jonas Robitscher labeled the "Power of Psychiatry." What *power* should the Supreme Court permit psychiatrists based on their expertise? Second, given that every citizen has a right to be left alone, how does mental illness negate or take away from that right? Third, what policies will the Supreme Court establish about the responsibilities of the states in meeting the needs of the mentally ill? Of these three questions, the last, the paternal obligations of the state, is the most political and possibly the most difficult to resolve. Judicial activists are willing to use the Constitution to force the states to meet the needs of the mentally disabled even if it means endless judicial intervention, social crisis, and expense, as has occurred in the area of school desegregation. Judicial conservatives, on the other hand, want to limit judicial activism, avoid legal intervention, and let legislators determine fiscal priorities. Both sides cite the Constitution to justify their policies and politics.

THE SECOND ILLUMINATION: GUESSING AND TRULY INFORMED GUESSING

Many psychiatrists, when they hear talk of the powers of psychiatry, immediately diagnose paranoia in the speaker. The everyday practice of psychiatry involves very little sense of power and a great deal of powerlessness in the face of human tragedy. But, as we say, there is a kernel of truth in paranoia. And in certain legal situations psychiatry does indeed have power.

The legal notion of insanity or mental incompetence wherever it occurs in law potentially gives power to psychiatry. Some critics suggest that no problem would be posed by writing the idea of insanity out of the law. But the law, for its own complicated reasons, resists doing so and the mental state of the individual is relevant in almost every area of law. For example, the law balks at the thought of executing an insane person. However, what the law means by the idea of insanity or incompetency in this and a variety of other legal contexts is quite ambiguous despite two centuries of attempts at developing precise legal definitions, and notwithstanding the recent application of the *Diagnostic and Statistical Manual of Mental Disorders*, Third Edition. This ambiguity permits psychiatrists to exercise considerable power—they are the ones called on by courts to give content to the term.

A powerful demonstration of what psychiatric power can mean can be seen in the 1950 Supreme Court case, *Solesbee v. Balkcom.*[3] Solesbee was a convicted murderer awaiting execution on death row in a Georgia prison; he claimed that he had become insane. The Governor of Georgia appointed a panel of three psychiatrists to examine Solesbee. These presumably impartial psychiatrists examined the man and by their own criteria and decision-making procedures diagnosed him as not insane and the Governor ordered his execution. (This approach of an appointed panel is similar to the Soviet approach described in the chapter on political misuse of psychiatry.)

It is worth considering for a moment what the role of psychiatry would have been if the panel *had* found Solesbee insane. Would some psychiatrist have had the obligation to establish a treatment relationship and restore Solesbee's sanity and reality testing so that he could be properly executed? This question is one of the many paradoxes in law and psychiatry.

In any event, Solesbee appealed to the Supreme Court, claiming he had a constitutional due-process right to a hearing on the question of his insanity. He wanted to offer his own psychiatric testimony, and he wanted to be able to cross-examine the presumably impartial psychiatrists who said he was sane. Justice Hugo Black, writing for the majority, rejected the due process claim on technical grounds having to do with the traditional authority of the Governor in matters of clemency. Presumably, the execution took place.

Ironically, the historical force of the case may stem from Justice Felix Frankfurter's vigorous dissent, in which he wrote that whether Solesbee was sane or insane was "in the present state of the mental sciences . . . at best a hazardous guess, . . . [a] life-and-death guess."[4] Justice Frankfurther concluded that, "[the] life-and-death guess will be a truly informed guess"[5] only if Solesbee was provided the basic ingredients of due process he requested.

The substantive significance between a guess and a truly informed guess was not spelled out by Frankfurter. But it is a difference that makes a great deal of difference to advocates of adversarial due process, such as Frankfurter. What Frankfurter had in mind was that when psychiatrists make a diagnosis of sanity or insanity behind their closed doors, it is only a guess. The law should not give power to psychiatry by enforcing such guesses. Only when the law opens the psychiatrists' doors and allows judge and jury to hear opposing counsel cross-examine psychiatrists can a truly informed guess be made.

Justice Frankfurter was not the first or the last Harvard lawyer to opine about the inadequacies of psychiatry. My colleague, Professor Alan Dershowitz, has asked, "Since psychiatrists cannot agree on what they are doing, isn't it better that they do it in open court?" This has been a basic plank for the past two decades in the constitutional movement to reform psychiatry. The due process remedy appeals to opponents of psychiatric power because in open court, (1) the psychiatrist's authority can be challenged, (2) legal conventions control the procedures for making the decision, and (3) the decision then becomes the ultimate responsibility of the court. We shall see what the Supreme Court thinks of this approach to truly informed guessing.

THE THIRD ILLUMINATION: THE SUPREME COURT IS AMBIVALENT

The Supreme Court, throughout its history, had never had the occasion to consider the constitutional implications of confining the mentally ill. Ironically, it was only when the mentally ill were charged with criminal offenses that the question of their constitutional rights was deemed worthy of the attention of the highest court. Thus, it seemed that the state could act with impunity in confining the mentally ill if they avoided pressing criminal charges or using quasi-criminal confinement (see Chapter 2, Psychiatry and Violence). The power of psychiatry, and the rights and needs of the mentally ill, had not been touched by the Constitution.

Justice Blackmun, in dealing with yet another case involving the rights of a "mentally ill" offender recognized this problem, and in 1972 it seemed that he spoke for the court when he addressed this striking omission and suggested that the Supreme Court was ready at last to remedy this neglect.

Jackson v. Indiana[6] was a very important case in its own right. It dealt with aspects of the legal questions discussed in the first chapter: competency to stand trial.

Theon Jackson was a 27-year-old deaf–mute with the intellectual capacities of a preschool child. Arrested for snatching the handbags of two women, Jackson was brought before an Indiana court, which invoked that state's procedures for determining a criminal defendant's competency to stand trial. The two psychiatrists who were appointed to examine Jackson concluded that he would not be able to participate in his own defense and that he was incapable of understanding the nature of the charges against him.

Upon receiving this report, the trial court committed Jackson to the care of the Indiana Department of Mental Health until such time as he could be certified as "sane." He was confined to a facility which had no staff person proficient in sign language. Jackson's counsel appealed— there had been no evidence presented that Jackson was insane, nor was there any hope that his mental abilities would improve so that he could be called sane, whatever that meant. Jackson was thus being committed to a "life sentence" without ever having been convicted of a crime. And he was being sent to a hospital that could not treat him.

This argument did not sway appellate courts within Indiana, but it proved convincing to the United States Supreme Court. Writing for a unanimous Court, Justice Blackmun agreed that Jackson's commitment without any formal hearing addressing his ability to function in society violated his equal protection and due process rights, and constituted unconstitutionally cruel and unusual punishment. He emphasized that the duration of confinement must bear some reasonable relationship to the purpose of confinement. This simple idea contained great promise. It presented a basic guideline for accountability; courts, it suggested, must look to the purpose of psychiatric confinements, at least in this context and perhaps in others.

On the way to reaching this conclusion, Justice Blackmun framed the larger issues in such a way that it seemed to denote a new awareness and interest on the high bench for clarifying the rights of the mentally ill. Discussing the traditionally broad power exercised by the states in committing the mentally ill, and noting the large number of persons affected, Blackmun wrote, "[I]t is . . . remarkable that the substantive constitutional limitations on this power have not been more frequently litigated."[7]

The very next line of the opinion, however, states, "We need not address these broad questions here,"[8] and it is this second line that anticipated the thrust of subsequent Supreme Court opinions. Although Justice Blackmun has himself attempted to pursue the rights of the mentally ill, his has often been a lone voice against denying petitions of certiorari in relevant cases. The Court has turned its back on the mentally ill. Although cases have reached the Supreme Court since *Jackson*, they have been dealt with in the narrowest possible way.

I have said that the Court is ambivalent, and I believe their ambivalence is based on a variety of conflicts. As already intimated, they are in conflict as a group. Solving the problems of the mentally ill is not an easy task, and some justices would prefer to leave this task to the states and the legislatures. Secondly, the Court's conservatives who want to avoid legal interventionism recognize that these cases are like Pandora's box. Once opened the legal ramifications are endless. Even if the Justices are concerned about the rights of the mentally ill, they do not want to pay this price. Thirdly, reading their opinions one gets the impression that they simply do not know what they want to do. They have no coherent policy and no clear direction. They have not even been willing to follow Justice Blackmun's simple guideline that the duration of confinement must bear a reasonable relationship to the purpose of confinement. They have been unable to sort out the legitimate purposes for confining the mentally ill.

It is characteristic of ambivalent persons that they cannot make up their minds, they practice denial and avoidance, they engage in obsessive ritual, they never get to the heart of the matter, they go round in circles, and they cannot take decisive action. They satisfy no one and they are themselves unsatisfied. The Supreme Court, of course, is not a person. I use ambivalence as a metaphor which captures the Court's dealings with the rights of the mentally ill. I shall try to demonstrate this when I describe what I have called the shell game of liberty and paternalism.

If the Supreme Court has been ambivalent, the lower federal courts have not been. They and many state courts have followed a policy which I describe in the next chapter. That policy is to restrict the "biased" discretionary authority of psychiatrists, to emphasize the autonomy of the alleged patient, and to require the states to meet the needs of the patients. These three goals are sometimes incompatible but the goals are clear.

THE FOURTH ILLUMINATION: LEGAL ABUSE OF PSYCHIATRIC POWER

The more the law has condemned psychiatric power, and the more it has criticized psychiatric expertise, the greater has been its demand for these discredited services. What is more, lawyers keep finding new uses for psychiatric testimony. The most dramatic example can be found in the area of capital punishment.

Capital punishment is the subject of one of this country's great moral debates. Polls show that a majority of Americans, increasingly fearful of the violence in society, now favor the death penalty. At an earlier time, when America's psychiatrists and the public were both more liberal than they are today, the APA submitted an *amicus curiae* (friend of the court) brief to the Supreme Court calling for the abolition of capital punishment. The brief was largely based on the work of UCLA psychiatrist Louis Jolyon West. It contained little in the way of legal argument; its main contention was that capital punishment was counterproductive as a deterrent. Justice Oliver Wendell Holmes once said, "I think that as life is action and passion, it is required of a man that he should share the passion and action of his time in peril of being judged not to have lived." The APA shared in the action and passion of the time against capital punishment, but the Supreme Court was not persuaded. In *Furman v. Georgia*,[9] although the Supreme Court vacated death sentences imposed under a Georgia statute essentially because of the statute's racially arbitrary administration, it suggested that if a fair, even-handed method for determining when to impose a death sentence could be developed, it would be held constitutional. Following this outline, some states have passed statutes under which psychiatrists have been given an important role in the determination of the sentence. After a verdict of guilt on a capital charge, psychiatrists for the prosecution and the defense can testify as to whether the defendant "would commit [future] criminal acts of violence that would constitute a continuing threat to society." Testimony is also relevant as to whether the defendant showed remorse.[10]

As I have already mentioned in discussing the ethics of forensic psychiatry, one psychiatrist in Texas has now testified in over 100 such death-penalty cases for the prosecution. An excellent participant in adversarial courtroom strategy, he gives similar convincing testimony in almost every case, diagnosing the defendant as an antisocial personality (a "sociopath" or "psychopath"). Since sociopaths do not learn from experience and show no remorse, they are essentially untreatable people who would certainly commit further criminal violence. The jury, after hearing this psychiatrist, almost never fails to impose the death penalty.

Judged by the Frankfurter standard, this psychiatrist is not exercising illegitimate power. His authority can be challenged, legal conventions control his testimony, and the ultimate decision is indeed left to the court. This psychiatrist is simply a skilled participant in the adversarial system, and it is to be expected that prosecuters will seek out his services. And as I have argued earlier, there is no clear ethical standard that he violates. However, there is much that is troubling about this testimony. Every empirical study has demonstrated that psychiatrists cannot make reliable long-term predictions of violence. The new Criminal Mental Health Standards proposed by the American Bar Association would not permit psychiatrists to testify as to future dangerousness. But these proposals have not yet been adopted by the ABA or enacted by any legislature.[11]

Taking a clue from Felix Frankfurter, the APA has advised the Supreme Court in amicus briefs that the prediction of future violence is a life-and-death guess, given the current state of mental science. The Supreme Court responded to these arguments in a case called Jurek v. Texas[12] by briefly noting the scientific evidence, but concluded that whether or not it was scientifically possible for psychiatrists and behavioral scientists to make such predictions, judges and juries make them every day.[13] The court's decision is reminiscent of the joke about the man who, when asked, "Do you believe in baptism?" answered, "Believe in it? Hell, I've seen it done!"

The APA has continued to press the argument about the scientific limitations of prediction. But in a subsequent case, *Estelle v. Smith*,[14] a different question arose: how does a psychiatrist obtain the information he or she uses to testify that defendants are incurable, dangerous sociopaths? The aforementioned Texas psychiatrist had examined a defendant named Smith before trial without informing him that the results of his examination might be the basis of testimony advocating his execution. The APA thought this was unethical and argued its unconstitutionality.

Whether the psychiatrist was acting ethically depends on what he knew at that time. Although it is clear that this psychiatrist often testified for the prosecution as to capital punishment, it is also clear that he often evaluated the competency of defendants in cases that did not reach a capital punishment stage. Thus he may not have known the uses to which his examination would be applied. To avoid these sorts of ethical problems, psychiatrists should always attempt to clarify the purpose and potential uses of their examinations before undertaking them. Further, they should lawfully resist unauthorized use of such examinations.

While the ethical questions in this case may have been ambiguous, the Court found that the constitutional questions were not. The Supreme Court held that Smith's Fifth Amendment right to remain silent and his Sixth Amendment right to effective counsel had been compromised by such a psychiatric examination. Justice Burger, who delivered the majority opinion in *Estelle*, commented in passing that some psychiatrists, citing me as an example, believe that psychiatrists possess no special qualifications for predicting future violence.[15] Nonetheless he emphasized that the Court expressed no disapproval of using psychiatric testimony.[16] However, after this case, prosecution psychiatrists were in the rather awkward position of being required to inform the defendant, and the defendant's lawyer, that the psychiatrist was conducting the examination for the purpose of testifying as to whether the defendant should be executed. This is certainly not the best way to establish rapport in psychiatric interviewing!

Prosecutors who have their own adversarial obligation to be zealous advocates developed an entirely new approach after *Estelle v. Smith*. As discussed in the chapter on the Ethical Boundaries of Forensic Psychiatry, in the case of one Thomas Barefoot, who was found guilty of murder, the psychiatrist took the stand at the sentencing phase to respond to a "hypothetical" scenario offered by the prosecutor. The hypothetical questions in effect summarized the defendant's criminal record and the testimony about the defendant's behavior offered during the trial. The psychiatrist, on the basis of the hypothetical questions gave his usual convincing testimony about dangerous psychopaths. The jury, persuaded by this testimony, sentenced the defendant, Barefoot, to death. Barefoot appealed and the case wound its way back and forth through federal and state courts.[17] It finally made its way to the Supreme Court with the APA in an *amicus* brief continuing its struggle to eliminate what it considered to be life-and-death guessing by psychiatrists. As I have already pointed out in the third chapter, in my view this testimony was not unethical by existing standards. The assertion of clinical certainty about future dangerousness is problematic and it is arguably unethical to claim such certainty in light of the empirical evidence; but I do not believe it is unethical for psychiatrists to answer hypothetical questions.

The Barefoot case involved other legal rulings which had important consequences for inmates of death row, but I shall discuss only the Court's resolution of the psychiatric testimony. The Fifth Circuit Court of Appeals had rejected the APA's arguments about prediction in much the same fashion as the Supreme Court had in *Jurek*: to accept such arguments would call into question all of the other legal contexts in which the prediction of future behavior is required by law. They mentioned the need for the jury to have "all possible relevant information,"[18] even when expert testimony may not be "totally accurate."[19] But the relevance of inaccurate expert testimony is, to say the least, problematic.

Justice White, writing for the Supreme Court's majority, was even more caustic about the APA's prediction arguments. He said the Court was being asked "to disinvent the wheel." It seemed ludicrous to him to bar psychiatric testimony as a matter of law and to allow lay testimony on the same issue. He echoed Frankfurter's view that the adversarial process could sort out the expert opinions. He emphasized the established role of predicting dangerousness in civil commitment. And throwing down the legal gauntlet to psychiatry, he argued that if the APA thought psychiatrists could not reliably predict dangerousness, then there should be no dearth of expert opinions to contradict the prosecution's experts. This, as we shall see, is also the law's answer in malpractice cases arising out of injuries to third parties.

Justice White also gave short shrift to the ethical or constitutional problems of psychiatrists answering hypothetical questions. That, he concluded, was an accepted and traditional practice under the rules of evidence. Justice Blackmun, citing the APA's *amicus* brief at great length, offered a vigorous dissent but to no avail. Justice White shrugged his opinion off as demonstrating a low evaluation of the adversary process.[20]

However, the APA *amicus* brief did not make what I consider to be the most important criticism of the psychiatric testimony. For the APA to have made that point would have required rejecting its own DSM-III and acknowledging DSM-III's social and racial bias. It would have meant exposing the value judgments in scientific objective psychiatry.

The invidious aspect of the testimony about sociopaths and their future dangerousness has to do with the racial and social implications of the diagnosis of sociopath as defined by DSM-III rather than with the ethics and expertise of the particular psychiatrists. The diagnostic criteria for antisocial personality in DSM-III might apply to the vast majority of those who face a death sentence as well as many black men who have grown up in inner cities. Those criteria include the following characteristics when manifest before age fifteen: (1) truancy, (2) delin-quency, (3) running away from home, (4) thefts, (5) vandalism, (6) school grades below expected, and (7) repeated sexual intercourse in a casual relationship. The existence of only three of these factors is sufficient to establish the disorder in this age group.

Over age eighteen, manifestations include (1) inability to sustain consistent work behavior, (2) lack of ability to function as a responsible parent, (3) failure to accept social norms, e.g. holding an illegal occupa-tion (pimping, prostitution, fencing, selling drugs), (4) inability to maintain enduring attachment to a sexual partner, (5) failure to honor financial obligations, (6) failure to plan ahead, (7) disregard for truth, and (8) recklessness. If there is a pattern of at least four such manifesta-tions, the diagnosis of sociopath is to be made.

Whatever scientific value the diagnosis of sociopath may have, there can be little question that the urban poor and racial minorities will be swept into this diagnostic category. DSM-III may well introduce the very racism the Supreme Court sought to eliminate in capital punish-ment cases. Even without the racial element, it should be noted that in most cases where the prosecution would press for execution, the defendant—black or white—would meet the DSM-III criteria of antiso-cial personality. Thus, the due process remedy and constitutional safeguards authored by the Supreme Court do not eliminate the abuse of psychiatric power in capital punishment cases, they just give it expres-sion in a new and possibly racist form.

THE FIFTH ILLUMINATION: THE SHELL GAME OF
LIBERTY AND PATERNALISM

I turn now to consider in more detail the Supreme Court's approach to the three policy questions: psychiatric power, autonomy, and paternalism. Mentally ill and mentally retarded persons who have committed no crimes have been confined under the most appalling conditions in state institutions for over a century. But it was not until 1975 that the Supreme Court considered a case dealing with the rights and needs of such patients.[21]

Kenneth Donaldson was a patient in Chatahoochee State Hospital in Florida. He had been committed on the petition of his father, who had become concerned about his son's "paranoid delusions."[22] It seems that Donaldson had told his father that he thought the neighbors might be poisoning him.[23] He may also have thought that his parents were poisoning him, and he once told a reporter that he had "blacked out" shortly before his first psychiatric hospitalization.[24] At the time of his commitment, Donaldson had been told by the judge that he would be in the hospital for "a few weeks."[25] In fact, he would remain there for fifteen years. Donaldson, claiming at times to be a Christian Scientist, refused to submit to electroshock treatment or treatment by medication, and he received no commonly accepted psychiatric treatment.[26] Donaldson's own view was that he was not mentally ill, and in fifteen legal petitions to various state and federal courts, he vainly sought his release. The courts apparently considered him just another *pro se* crank and ignored and rejected his legal efforts. Mr. Donaldson—who has since written a book, appeared on television, and lectured at various colleges about his experience—is clearly an articulate and literate man. But between 1957 and 1972, he got no help from the federal courts in spite of his invoking a wide range of constitutional provisions, including the writ of *habeas corpus* and various due process attacks on his confinement.

Dr. O'Connor, the psychiatrist responsible for his care, had diagnosed Mr. Donaldson as a chronic paranoid schizophrenic, and as psychiatrists are apt to do, he interpreted Donaldson's various legal attempts to obtain his freedom as symptoms of litigious paranoia. Dr. O'Connor, exercising his discretionary power under law, responded to this litigious paranoia by setting therapeutic limits on Mr. Donaldson: denying him grounds privileges, confining him to a ward for the criminally insane, and stopping Mr. Donaldson's "occupational therapy" because there Mr. Donaldson could use a typewriter to prepare legal briefs and to draft letters to various newspapers depicting his situation and the dreadful conditions at Chatahoochee State Hospital. There is also evidence that Dr. O'Connor interfered with plans for Mr. Donaldson's release to various caretakers who offered to help, on the theory that the people who were willing to assume responsibility for such a difficult litigious patient as Donaldson should not be taken seriously.

During Donaldson's confinement, Dr. O'Connor typically had as many as six hundred to one thousand other patients under his care. He rarely spoke to Donaldson, whom he considered merely a paranoid patient with a poor prognosis who took up more than his fair share of time by causing aggravation and administrative paperwork. Donaldson was one squeaky wheel who was not going to get greased, or so Dr. O'Connor apparently thought at the time. (I have no reason to believe that Dr. O'Connor acted in bad faith. We discussed the case and his management of it several times by telephone, through which it became apparent that he viewed the state hospital as a provider of custodial care for chronic mental patients. The community mental health approach, the revolving door, and deinstitutionalization were not being practiced between 1957 and 1972 by the administrators of Chatahoochee State Hospital.)

How Mr. Donaldson finally got his day in federal court is an interesting tale. Unable to find a lawyer who would be interested in helping him to obtain his freedom and his autonomy, Donaldson finally contacted Dr. Morton Birnbaum, the spiritual father of the right-to-treatment movement. Dr. Birnbaum, perhaps because he is a general practitioner of medicine and a lawyer only on the side, believes in paternalism. He believes that the states have a moral, medical, and constitutional obligation to provide humane treatment in state mental hospitals. His efforts have been devoted to giving real substance to the states' hypocritical shell game of supposed paternalism. Warehousing people in degrading conditions, as has happened to hundreds of thousands of mentally ill and mentally retarded persons, is not paternalism, nor is depriving people of liberty, supposedly in order to help them, only to ignore, neglect, and abuse them. His goal was not to close the state hospitals but rather to improve the quality of care available in them.

If I am overstating the views I impute to Dr. Birnbaum, it is because I share with him a strong belief that society has failed to allocate the necessary resources to deal with the problems of the mentally ill and retarded. This failure in our basic human obligations must be confronted. Often, attacking psychiatry and paternalism in the name of autonomy only serves as a distraction from the real issue, providing adequate resources for humane care. Even if this is so, the question remains whether it is proper, given the doctrine of separation of powers, to expect the federal courts to use their power to force the states to meet these human obligations. Using any particular court case to confront general societal issues can present anomalies, as the *Donaldson* case illustrates.

Dr. Birnbaum and Mr. Donaldson made a very strange pair. Mr. Donaldson wanted to get out of Chatahoochee, insisting that he was not mentally ill and needed no treatment. He was, and is, an advocate of the "alleged" patients' right to be left alone. His lawyer, Dr. Birnbaum, however, was an advocate of paternalism. He wanted to require the State of Florida to improve the conditions and the quality of treatment of "real" patients in what was a grossly understaffed and inadequate state hospital.

Lawyer and client reconciled their interests, but only at the cost of creating considerable confusion in the courts. Dr. Birnbaum's original legal complaint spoke directly to two of the main policy questions which have concerned the Supreme Court. First, the case was a class action in which the court was asked to release Donaldson and all the other patients in his section of the hospital. Thus, Donaldson's autonomy claim was asserted. But they were to be released because they were not getting treated, not because they had a right to be left alone.

Second, Birnbaum argued that there was a constitutional right to treatment and he asked the court to order massive improvements in the section of the hospital from which Donaldson and the others were to be released. Thus, Dr. Birnbaum was asserting his own interest in paternalism by asking the court to grapple with the blatantly political question of how much treatment resources a court could order a state to supply.

By the time the trial took place in federal court, a great deal had changed. Dr. O'Connor had retired with a heart condition. The doctors who took his place had discharged Mr. Donaldson, and Dr. Birnbaum himself had been replaced by two trial lawyers. Dr. Birnbaum's original complaint was severed and amended. In the end, all that remained was a damage action against Dr. O'Connor for exercising his power under color of law to deprive Mr. Donaldson of his constitutional rights. This "1983 action,"[27] as it is known to lawyers, was an attack on the discretionary power of psychiatrists in their management of patients in the hospital.

The crucial question at trial was to determine precisely which constitutional right Mr. Donaldson had been deprived of by Dr.

O'Connor. The jury heard testimony from psychiatrists who, unlike Dr. O'Connor, would have dealt with a chronic paranoid patient not with custodial care but by facilitating his discharge as quickly as possible. Under that standard Dr. O'Connor's use of his discretionary authority was terrible. The best treatment would have been to release Mr. Donaldson to a halfway house, but Dr. O'Connor had rejected such a plan in a way that in restrospect seemed malicious. The jury's verdict including punitive damages was that Dr. O'Connor wantonly and maliciously deprived Mr. Donaldson of his constitutional right to treatment. That answer came as quite a surprise because at the time only one federal judge, Alabama District Court Judge Frank Johnson, in the landmark case of *Wyatt v. Stickney*, had held that the right to treatment could be found in the Constitution.[28]

In *Wyatt*, which preceded *Donaldson*, Judge Johnson had ordered Governor Wallace and the State of Alabama to spend millions of dollars to put something real under the empty shell of paternalism. Alabama had by all accounts the worst public mental institutions in the country, and the documented indignities to patients which were revealed at the trial should shock the conscience of any human being. Nonetheless, Alabama appealed to the Fifth Circuit claiming that (1) there was no right to treatment under the Constitution, (2) if there were such a right, it was non-justiciable (a matter judges were incapable of deciding), and (3) under the Eleventh Amendment, the federal courts did not have the power to reorder state fiscal priorities as they have been established through state legislative decision-making. The Fifth Circuit for two years had delayed action on Alabama's appeal, and it was widely rumored that a majority could not be found for Judge Johnson's courageous political decision and judicial activism.

The Florida Attorney General, representing Dr. O'Connor, appealed *Donaldson* to the Fifth Circuit while that court was sitting on *Wyatt*. Echoing Alabama's arguments in *Wyatt*, Florida asserted that there was no constitutional right to treatment and, therefore, Dr. O'Connor could not be liable for depriving Mr. Donaldson of a nonexistent right. The *Donaldson* case differed from *Wyatt*, though, because it did not directly confront the political question. *Donaldson* did not require the state of Florida to spend millions of dollars on its state hospitals. The jury had awarded Mr. Donaldson approximately $28,000, including $10,000 in punitive damages. *Donaldson* did not require judicial activism and interventionism in the sense that a federal court had to invoke the Constitution to tell the states how to run all of their mental institutions. The power of federal judges was not pitted against that of state officials. The case did not seek to remedy the real deficiencies of state institutions. Rather, it merely sought to vindicate one patient's claim against his psychiatrist's discretionary authority.

With the issues framed in that manner, the Fifth Circuit had no difficulty finding the right to treatment in the Constitution.[29] While Florida was appealing *Donaldson* to the Supreme Court, the Fifth Circuit boldly decided *Wyatt* on the precedent it had just set in *Donaldson*.[30] In the due process clause of the Fourteenth Amendment, the court saw the foundation for a "two-part theory" of the right to treatment.[31] The first part consists of the view that any nontrivial abridgment of freedom must serve some permissible governmental goal. One such goal, the court agreed, is the paternalistic provision of treatment, but only if treatment is in fact provided. Thus, those committed for the purpose of treatment have a right to treatment. The second part of the theory is that confinement imposed without compliance with all relevant constitutional limitations must be accompanied by a *quid pro quo* (something given in exchange for something else). Rehabilitative treatment is the most appropriate *quid pro quo* for confinement of the mental patient who has committed no specific offense, is confined for no fixed term, and is detained without full procedural safeguards. Thus, the court concluded, those confined under such circumstances have a right to treatment. Relying on this reasoning in *Donaldson*, the Fifth Circuit upheld Judge Johnson's judicial activism and the massive decrees against the State of Alabama.

Implementing Judge Johnson's decree has not been easy. Twelve years have passed and Alabama has still not fully complied with the order of the court. *Donaldson* had gotten the camel's nose in the tent, and with *Wyatt*, the entire animal of judicial activism and interventionism had pushed its way in, but a real solution to the problems raised by the cases has not yet been found.

Finding receptive circuit court judges is one thing, but convincing the Supreme Court is another matter, and it was to the Supreme Court that Florida had turned. The lawyers who argued for Donaldson knew that Chief Justice Burger, an avowed opponent of judicial activism, including the finding of new substantive constitutional rights, would likely oppose the right to treatment. Burger would no doubt attempt to use the *Donaldson* case as an opportunity to throw the camel out of the tent. The lawyers, knowing that it would be difficult to get full approval of a right to treatment from what was in 1975 an increasingly conservative Supreme Court, adroitly shuffled the shells and put *Donaldson* under the one marked "Liberty." Autonomy, not paternalism, became the issue. Under this approach, what was important was only that Dr. O'Connor had used his power under the law to deprive

Donaldson of his constitutional liberty. The facts of Donaldson's case lent credence to this legal strategy because the effective treatment urged for him was that he be released. The right to treatment and the right to autonomy were in Donaldson's case identical. But if this strategy was helpful to the cause of civil libertarians it may have been less helpful to Donaldson's claim for damages. All of the courts passing judgment on this issue had themselves rejected Donaldson's prior attempts to secure his freedom. How could one blame Dr. O'Connor for acting in bad faith when the responsible courts had taken the same action? Chief Justice Burger would emphasize this in his opinion, but he was outfoxed on the constitutional right to treatment.

He was denied the opportunity to throw the camel out entirely. A majority of the court in fact agreed with his rejection of the right to treatment.[32] Unfortunately for the Chief Justice, they also agreed with Donaldson that he had been seriously wronged. Thinking he had a majority behind him, Burger wrote an opinion condemning the right to treatment.[33] Dissatisfied with his failure to condemn the circumstances of Donaldson's lengthy confinement, Burger's colleagues on the Supreme Court simply ignored the right to treatment and found what they wanted under the liberty shell: the state could not continue to confine a mentally ill person who was not dangerous to himself or others, who was not being treated, and who could survive outside the hospital. Justice Burger's argument was reduced to the status of a concurring opinion.

But what, you may ask, happened to the Fifth Circuit's right to treatment precedent, which had been applied through Wyatt? In a remarkable footnote, the Supreme Court explained that their decision deprived the Court of Appeal's opinion of precedential effect.[34] Legally this meant that Wyatt was res judicata but not stare decisis: the Wyatt decision would stand, but it was technically not to be used as a precedent for other similar cases. This technicality seems to have detracted little from the legal importance of Wyatt.

Only Donaldson's damage judgment against Dr. O'Connor was left unsettled by the Supreme Court, which remanded this issue to the Fifth Circuit, which in turn sent the question back to the Florida District Court where it was finally settled out of court. Mr. Donaldson, who had been confined for fifteen years in a snake pit, ended up with a mere $20,000, half for his claim against the then deceased Dr. O'Connor and half for his claim against another doctor. With only a trace of bitterness, Donaldson wryly once mentioned to me that by comparison, the federal courts had required the State of Florida to pay more than half a million dollars to the lawyers who had replaced Dr. Birnbaum.

Mr. Donaldson interpreted the Supreme Court's decision as proving that he was not mentally ill. Civil libertarians saw *Donaldson* as a
great victory for the autonomy of alleged mental patients and against the
discretionary power of psychiatry to decide on psychiatric grounds who
belongs in a mental hospital. In fact the courts reached neither of these
results. The very narrow holding, speaks only to the one question of
when a mental patient must be released. Again, despite this technical
description of the narrowness of the holding, the opinion has since been
read by judges the same way civil libertarians read it. However one
might interpret the decision, it seemed to me the Court, even by its
narrow holding, was creating another incentive (the danger of a damage
action) for states to avoid their paternal responsibilities by discharging
chronic patients into the community. I was not surprised, therefore,
when New York State's Commissioner of Mental Health announced
that in light of the Supreme Court's decision, he was prepared to
convert all chronic patients to voluntary status and allow them to leave
the hospital. The bag lady is, for me, a symbol of the Supreme Court's
Donaldson decision. Mr. Donaldson did not need paternalism, but there
are many people who do.

Chief Justice Burger, in a blistering concurring opinion in
Donaldson, did seize the opportunity at least to polemicize against the
Fifth Circuit's constitutional *quid pro quo* theory of the right to
treatment. His argument had two prongs which pointed in opposite
directions. First he defended the states' authority to provide custodial
care without treatment, suggesting that he was not concerned about the
liberty or the treatment of mental patients as a constitutional matter.
Then, as an apparent defender of the patient's liberty, the essence of his
argument was first that there was no deprivation of due process and
second that due process could not be altered as the *quo* for any *quid*.
Thus he rejected this or any other theory of the right to treatment. He
wrote, "I . . . can discern no basis for equating an involuntarily committed mental patient's unquestioned constitutional right not to be confined without due process of law with a constitutional right to
treatment."[35] The essence of his argument was first that there was no
deprivation of due process and second that due process could not be
altered as the *quo* for any *quid*. Thus he rejected this or any other theory
of the right to treatment. The judges in the lower courts have by no
means been cowed by the Chief Justice, and since 1975, with ingenious
lawyers pushing litigation all over the country, the right to treatment
has led a herd of camels into the tent.

In the wake of the *Donaldson* "victory," there followed a series of

Supreme Court cases in which civil libertarians sought to extend due process reform to psychiatry. These cases exposed the court's ambivalence as earlier described. In *Addington v. Texas*,[36] the Supreme Court was asked to rule that the Constitution required that states must satisfy the "beyond a reasonable doubt" evidentiary standard before a person could be civilly committed. As precedent, the Supreme Court was directed to look to its own opinion in a case involving the confinement of juveniles, in which the criminal justice "beyond a reasonable doubt" standard was required.[37]

This technical legal question of the standard of proof had important consequences. There are three common standards, which in increasing levels of exactitude are (1) the "preponderance of the evidence" standard, (2) the "clear and convincing evidence" standard, and (3) the "beyond a reasonable doubt" standard.

The growing legal consensus that psychiatry is guesswork which must be sifted through the adversarial context creates problems for law itself, problems which tend to increase the courts' ambivalence. Civil libertarians would argue that when loss of liberty is at stake, the government should be made to prove its case beyond a reasonable doubt. We have already seen the problems that the "beyond a reasonable doubt" standard created in the insanity trial of John Hinckley; similar problems arise in ordinary civil commitment. If psychiatry is guesswork, how can the state in an adversarial hearing prove beyond a reasonable doubt that someone is mentally ill and dangerous? Yet civil commitment clearly involves a loss of liberty, so civil libertarians argue that the state must do the impossible by proving its case beyond a reasonable doubt. Recognizing the impossibility of proving mental illness and dangerousness beyond a reasonable doubt, civil libertarians have urged a past-act requirement, which involves an act of violence or a clear threat of violence. The past act or threat can be proved beyond a reasonable doubt in exactly the same way that courts make such determinations in criminal cases. But many states do not have a past-act requirement and yet require proof beyond a reasonable doubt. Courts either must pretend that psychiatry is not guesswork or they must require a past act in practice even when the statute does not. Civil libertarians prefer the latter alternative. But whatever the courts' practices may be with a "beyond a reasonable doubt" standard, they have firmer ground on which to attack the psychiatric guesswork. But the Supreme Court neither accepted the civil libertarian argument nor followed the expected precedent. Justice Marshall asked during oral argument, "Do you think psychiatrists can prove anything beyond a reasonable doubt?" In the spirit of that question the Supreme Court held that the Constitution required only clear and convincing evidence.

Then, in *Parham v. J.R.*, the majority took a position directly against the trend of due process reforms I described earlier as the basic plank of civil libertarian reform. The question confronted was what due process were children entitled to when, with a psychiatrist's approval, their parents or a state agency placed them in mental institutions. Civil libertarians, of course, demanded due process hearings with lawyers for the children, cross-examination of parents and psychiatrists, and ulti- mate decision-making power confined solely to a judge.

Justice Burger, writing for the majority, turned his back on the Frankfurter approach to due process and "truly informed guessing," writing, "although we acknowledge the fallibility of medical and psychiatric diagnosis . . . we do not accept the notion that the short- comings of specialists can always be avoided by shifting the decision from a trained specialist using the traditional tools of medical science to an untrained judge . . . after a judicial-type hearing,"[38] adding "the supposed protections of an adversary hearing . . . may well be more illusory than real"[39]

Was Justice Burger bowing to the expertise of psychiatry? The APA thought so, feeling a great initial sense of satisfaction. But I think we misunderstood. Justice Burger does not have a higher opinion of our expertise than did Justice Frankfurter. Justice Burger is simply opposed to judicial interventionism. His support of psychiatry was merely his way of demonstrating that. Psychiatry was only a pawn in the politics of the court. *Parham* produced howls of protest from civil libertarians, and even I was unhappy with the result, though for different reasons.

Whether a child is given due process or not, it is inexcusable to send a child to a degrading, dehumanizing institution that masquerades as a hospital. This is and was the real issue in *Parham*, and the Supreme Court was evading it. And of course, the same concerns apply to adults. The *Parham* case had come from Georgia, a state in which the facilities for children were terrible. A Commission appointed by the Governor of Georgia had come to that conclusion in a report in response to which the state had failed to act. The lower court had recognized the real horror of the situation, and their decision, although disguised in the language of due process, was meant to force the state to adopt a policy of providing alternative and better treatment facilities for children. The decision in fact quoted at length from the Commission report. They were invoking due process to obtain better care for children. They recognized that the problem was not the discretionary power of parents or psychiatrists but the lack of necessary services. This was the case in which Justice Stewart wrote the line I quoted earlier as my First Illumination. Ironically, however, Justice Stewart made no mention of the terrible institutions documented in the lower court's decision. Instead, the policy issue that concerned him involved the rights of parents, who might be unfit to decide what was in their children's best interests. But it was our mental institutions which were actually unfit, and the Supreme Court would eventually be forced to face that fact.

The most recent manifestation of the Court's view of psychiatry as guesswork and their own ambivalence came in the case of *Jones v. United States*.[40] Jones, who was charged with attempted petit larceny following his arrest for trying to steal a jacket from a department store, was diagnosed as a paranoid schizophrenic, although he was deemed competent to stand trial. Jones' plea of not guilty by reason of insanity was unopposed by the government, and, pursuant to District of Columbia statutory law, he was committed to St. Elizabeth's Hospital following the court's acceptance of his plea. The trouble was that the commitment of an insanity acquittee required proof of insanity by only a preponderance of evidence, the lowest standard of evidence possible, while the Court in *Addington* had required proof by clear and convincing evidence for civil commitment. Jones argued that he should be released unless the government could commit him under the higher standard. The Supreme Court rejected that argument, explaining that the higher standard was designed to ensure against commitments based on "mere idiosyncratic behavior," and that in insanity acquittal cases, such idiosyncratic commitments were prevented by the finding that the defendant had committed a crime, that is, a past act. Of course in Jones' case, the past act was shoplifting—not a very convincing basis in the first place for assuming Jones was dangerous.

The real problem of course is that the Court has no coherent policy about the rights of the mentally ill. Unable to solve the legal problems rationally, the Justices make dubious and ambivalent arguments about the standard of proof.

THE FINAL ILLUMINATION: THE SUPREME COURT IS NOT THAT IMPORTANT

In short order, the Justices were confronted with two cases which revealed the unfitness of institutions for the mentally retarded. The first case was a class action initiated in 1974 challenging the constitutionality of conditions at the Pennhurst State School and Hospital, a Pennsylvania facility for the mentally retarded. The Federal Court heard undisputed testimony establishing just how dangerous Pennhurst was: residents were frequently physically abused or inappropriately drugged by staff members; few efforts were made to "habilitate" residents of the hospital; and the physical, intellectual, and emotional status of many of the residents in fact deteriorated during their stay at the hospital. Much the same testimony could be given about many institutions for the mentally retarded across the United States. The federal district court trying this case held that Pennhurst's mentally retarded residents

> (1) had a federal constitutional right to be provided with "minimally adequate habilitation" in the "least restrictive environment," (2) were being subject to cruel and unusual punishment in violation of the Eighth Amendment and were being discriminated against in violation of the Fourteenth Amendment equal protection clause; and (3) had statutory rights under federal and state funding laws providing for the care of the retarded.[41]

Having invoked these rights, the court took a costly and interventionist approach and ordered that suitable community living arrangements be found for all Pennhurst residents, with individual treatment plans developed with family participation. The court mandated that conditions at Pennhurst be improved until the court's order could be fully carried out and Pennhurst closed completely. A Special Master was appointed to oversee implementation of the court's order.

On appeal,[42] the Third Circuit confined the lower court's ruling to its statutory basis only and vacated altogether that part of the order calling for the total closing of Pennhurst, demanding instead that the court or the Special Master make individual considerations for each present or future resident. But the Third Circuit generally approved of the highly activist decision, taking no steps to lessen the intervention of a federal court in its takeover of the administration of a state facility. This was a very important practical matter. As Judge Johnson had found in *Wyatt*, it was no easy matter to get the state to do what the court ordered. Here the court had taken the bold step of giving an order and appointing the Special Master to carry out that order.

The Third Circuit avoided reaching a constitutional right to habilitation (habilitation is treatment in the retardation context) by finding sufficient basis for the holding in various provisions of the Federal Developmentally Disabled Assistance and Bill of Rights Act[43] (hereinafter referred to as "DDABRA"), in particular the DDABRA's "Bill of Rights" provision, which articulated the ideal of granting to the mentally retarded "appropriate treatment, services, and habilitation," in a setting "that is least restricting of . . . personal liberty."[44] By pointing to a legislative basis for its decision, the court was able to affirm the lower court decision without seeming to affirm judicial intervention‐ ism—the intervention had come from the legislative branch in the form of statutory law. Still, the court had imposed an expensive burden on the states, and that was enough for the three dissenters on the court to view the decision as improperly interventionistic.

The Supreme Court, when first faced with *Pennhurst*, totally evaded expressing an opinion on the substantive issues in the case, reversing the circuit court opinion on its interpretation of the federal statute, but remanding the case for reconsideration under state law. Writing for the Court, Justice Rehnquist declared he could "find nothing in the act or its legislative history to suggest that Congress intended to require the states to assume the high cost of providing 'appropriate treatment' in a 'least restrictive environment.'"[45] The Bill of Rights provision, he ruled, was merely there to "assist" states, expressing only a congressional "preference for a certain kind of treatment."[46] Justice Rehnquist reasoned that if Congress had intended to mandate rather than merely encourage such a radical treatment reform model, it would have provided much more than the 1.6 million dollars of federal money allocated to Pennsylvania under the Act in 1976.

It is possible to debate Justice Rehnquist's reading of the legislative history. Such readings are one of the great mysteries of the highest bench. Having participated in the legislative process, Senator Javits of New York would certainly reject Rehnquist's reading. But if one asks whether Congress knew when they voted for DDABRA that the Bill of Rights provision would be used to force the states to do what the lower court in *Pennhurst* required, the answer would probably be no. Perhaps Congress was tossing the hot potato to the courts, saying, "let the courts tell us what we mean." Rehnquist's decision can be defended by judicial conservatives on the grounds that it tells the legislature to take responsibility for these major policy decisions, and that, after all, is the proper role of a legislature in our government.

On remand, the circuit court was not backing off when they cited independent state grounds to support their earlier decision—in the interim the Pennsylvania Supreme Court had ruled that a Pennsylvania funding statute did require the least restrictive alternative consistent with adequate treatment and care. Several members of the circuit court questioned the role of the Master, though, arguing that a federal court had to assume that a state would comply with a federal court order and that the federal court should do no more than state what would constitute compliance with the law and leave it up to the state to comply or forego federal funding. One judge wrote that in any event courts should not decide which patients go where. "Individual medical decisions . . . must be left to the judgment of physicians in each case."[47]

The Supreme Court has at this writing again heard an appeal of the circuit court ruling,[48] but has yet to decide. As before, there are many ways the Supreme Court could avoid reaching the substantive issues. Ample technical loose ends have been laid bare by the various opinions. The Court could easily render a very narrow, highly legalistic decision based on Eleventh Amendment principles of federalism, standing to sue, or the role of a Master, etc. They might ask and answer a very complicated question: why is a federal court enforcing a state law instead of a state court?

In the meantime, the case continues to bounce around the lower federal courts. While the Supreme Court cautiously deliberates, Pennhurst is slowly being emptied of its residents at great cost to the state, and the court's involvement, through the Master, in making individual determinations about retarded patients, creates the constant potential of litigation. One such suit has already reached the Third Circuit resulting in a ruling which might in fact be a precedential time bomb capable of undermining much of the prior progress made by the lawsuit. In *Halderman v. Pennhurst*, a voluntarily committed, profoundly retarded minor at Pennhurst was ordered by the district court to be transferred to a community living arrangement.[49] The district court had adopted the report of the Master who followed all of the correct procedures, including the use of parental input, to reach the conclusion that this decision was in the best interests of the child. But the child's parents contested the transfer. They wanted their child to stay at Pennhurst and argued that their constitutional parental rights were being violated by the transfer order. Once more they were confronting the *Parham* question: what authority do parents have in deciding the question of what is in the best interest of their children?

The Third Circuit held that neither the Master nor the district court had made any factual or procedural errors, but the Constitution "mandates a judicial obligation to respect, if not protect, parental authority and decisions relating to general family matters."[50] The issue, according to the Third Circuit, was whether the state had "demon-strated a sufficiently important interest to justify governmental interference with the parental decision making authority," citing various prominent freedom of religion cases, abortion cases, and the *Parham* case.[51]

Parham, as they interpreted it, held that the parents' right to have their child voluntarily committed could be subordinated to either the child's basic liberty interest in not being unnecessarily confined or the state's significant interest in maintaining control over the utilization of its facilities. The Third Circuit read this to mean that the parents did have a "substantial" constitutional right, but not a "fundamental" constitutional right, to "direct and control the upbringing and develop-ment of their minor children. . . . Absent a showing of abuse and neglect, the parental right . . . may be subject to governmental interfer-ence only when such interference is supported by significant govern-mental interests."[52]

The Third Circuit ruled that because of this parental constitu-tional right, the burden of proving the necessity of the transfer thus lay on the government, which must show abuse or neglect, and that the treatment being accorded to the "child" at Pennhurst was equivalent to abuse or neglect. Since the evidence concerning what would be a preferable placement was conflicting—witnesses called by the parents and the state disagreed with one another—the parents should have been given a substantial, if not dominant, role in the final decision, the court held.

As Judge Sloviter noted in his dissent, a decision to transfer a child back to Pennhurst over a finding by the Master that the community living arrangement was more beneficial could eviscerate all of the earlier *Pennhurst* holdings.[53] How could the court overrule the procedures it had previously approved, and how could it declare Pennhurst to be an adequate treatment facilty without jeopardizing all of the earlier suits? These concerns may be exaggerated. Presumably many parents will agree with the Master's decisions which have already been imple-mented. But the decision does suggest the kind of problem which has now arisen in class action suits like *Pennhurst*. In some instances parents and families will agree with legal advocates pressing for massive deinstitutionalization under the least restrictive alternative. However, in other cases, families have concluded that community placements are problematic—for example, they are difficult to oversee and supervise, promising programs may not be lasting programs, and the state facility is more permanent and more tangible (that is, it is sure to be there when the parents are gone). It is one thing for a federal judge to empty a facility like Pennhurst when the experts, the families, and the legal advocates all are giving the same message. But when the messages are mixed, so are the judicial readings of what the Constitution requires. It remains to be seen how the Supreme Court will deal with these issues in the future. But as indicated by *Youngberg v. Romeo*, the most significant decision in this area, even the Justices of the Supreme Court cannot turn their backs on extreme instances of neglect.

In *Youngberg*, the Court took the tiniest steps toward responsible paternalism.[54] Nicholas Romeo, a mentally retarded 33yearold man with an IQ equivalent to that of a typical 1½yearold child, had been cared for by his parents at home until his father died. His mother, unable to deal with Nicholas by herself or manage his violence, turned to the state for help, and Nicholas was "committed" to an institution. Nicholas' needs for care were enormous and the state failed in its paternalistic responsibilities. Once in the institution, he "suffered injuries" on at least 63 occasions and was repeatedly placed in restraints for long periods of time. Like Donaldson, he sued for damages and claimed that he had been denied his constitutional right to habilitation.

At trial, the defendants won a jury verdict and judgment in their favor. However, the district court had excluded from the trial expert testimony concerning the circumstances surrounding Romeo's injuries, and it had given the jury instruction based on a questionable theory of the rights of mentally retarded inmates. These served as the principal grounds for appeal. The Third Circuit Court of Appeals vacated the lower court judgment and remanded for a new trial. In doing so the court set out a complex theory of the rights of the mentally retarded. Each aspect of an inmate's situation was to be evaluated by a different standard. Shackling, for example, would be acceptable only if justified by a "compelling necessity" and only if a no less restrictive method of dealing with an inmate was available. Determination of whether these standards were met was to be left to the jury.[55]

Furthermore, the court held that only a "substantial necessity" would justify failure to protect an inmate from attack.[56] This was apparently regarded by the court as a higher standard than that of compelling necessity; again, a jury was to decide whether the condition was met. A right to treatment was also recognized by the court. This right was based on due process requirements related to the purpose of confinement—that is, treatment—and the court held that in a case such as Romeo's, the right required the provision of treatment which could be regarded as acceptable for him in light of present medical or other scientific knowledge.[57] This ruling was appealed. The Supreme Court was thus faced with another interventionist opinion, one which made

the courts the primary decision makers on many aspects of care of the retarded and one which could impose great costs on the states.

Justice Powell, who had sided with Rehnquist in the *Pennhurst*
decision, analyzed Romeo's situation in terms of his " 'historic liberty
interest' protected substantively by the due process clause."[58] He made
much of the fact that Romeo had been committed. In fact, Romeo had
been placed in a state institution because there was no other place
which could care for him. The state had no interest in depriving Romeo
of his liberty, and he had no meaningful way to exercise his liberty. But
having established that right, the Court found some paternalism under
the shell of liberty. Justice Powell reached paternalism by supporting
Romeo's constitutional liberty right to be free from unsafe conditions
and undue physical restraints.

The majority concluded that Romeo's liberty interests required the
state to provide minimally adequate or reasonable training, but only to
the extent necessary to insure his safety and allow him freedom from
undue restraint. The Court carefully qualified this substantive due
process right under the Fourteenth Amendment. They deferred to the
experts in deciding what was reasonable, cautioning against judicial
intervention, and again avoided the question of whether there is a *per se*
right to treatment. Justice Powell deftly sidestepped this issue by noting
that Romeo's attorneys had conceded that no amount of training would
make his release possible, and the record showed that his *primary* needs
concerned his bodily safety and freedom from restraint. Justice Powell
was thus able to question whether Romeo was even asking for any
habilitation unrelated to safety, allowing him to conclude that "this case
does not present the difficult question whether a mentally retarded
person, involuntarily committed to a state institution, has some general
constitutional right to training *per se*."[59] Justice Powell couldn't resist
one small free bite at the issue, noting that "professionals in the
habilitation of the mentally retarded disagree strongly on the question
whether effective training of all severely or profoundly retarded individuals is even possible."[60]

Justice Blackmun concurred with the majority, but he was not
quite as convinced about the underlying constitutional grounds. Justice
Blackmun noted that due process "might well bind the state to insure
that the conditions of . . . [a] commitment bear some reasonable relation
to [its] goals, (the language he had used in Jackson). In such a case,
commitment without any 'treatment' whatsoever would not bear a
reasonable relation to the purposes of the person's confinement."[61]

Only Chief Justice Burger was willing to address the issue

squarely. He wrote that he "would hold flatly that respondent has no constitutional right to . . . 'habilitation.' . . . [The] Constitution does not . . . place an affirmative duty on the state to provide any particular kind of training or habilitation."[62]

Reading the opinions, it is sometimes hard to keep in mind how the cases got started—who the plaintiffs really are, what these institutions are really like, and what therapy and habilitation can and cannot do for people with these illnesses or conditions. If I were responsible for Romeo's care, I would have no practical idea about what was in fact required by the Constitution. There are limited resources in any institution; does the Constitution require that the most severely retarded like Romeo have first priority in training to insure their safety and freedom? If the only means of achieving his safety and freedom is twenty-four hour personal attendants, must the institution supply that? It is totally unclear what counts as meeting Romeo's constitutional right. But maybe this is precisely the point. The Supreme Court's majority is no longer trying to solve these difficult problems; rather they are avoiding them in any way they can. The Justices are caught up in their subjective notions of the role of the judiciary in the modern federalist state. Issues like the right to treatment of the mentally retarded or the mentally ill become vehicles for allowing each Justice to espouse his or her particular political theories regarding the meaning of constitutional phrases and the role of the federal courts in our horizontal and vertical separation-of-powers schema.

The irony of this—which demonstrates my last illumination, that the Supreme Court is not that important—is that Romeo is a patient in Pennhurst. Pennhurst is the institution being cleared out by a Master appointed by the lower federal court under the most expansive theory of the right to treatment imaginable; namely, the right to treatment in the least restrictive alternative. The Master, as we have seen, is completely ignoring the Supreme Court's cautions about intervention, and even the circuit court, when it has overruled the decision of the Master, has deferred not to the state but rather to parents. The federal court has forced the state to come up with the necessary funds to finance their intervention through the Master, and when the state has balked, the court has held state officials in contempt to the tune of ten thousand dollars a day, thereby collecting the necessary funds to support the Master's interventions.

The actual battle over such issues as the scope of the right to treatment is thus still being carried out on a daily level by patient advocates, families, the hospitals, and the state mental health bureaucracies prodded by the lower federal courts. Without the Supreme Court's blessing, federal courts all across the country are moving ahead, and it seems to me the Supreme Court has neither the will to stop them nor the willingness to encourage them.

Over the last few years I have discussed these cases with many federal judges. Some are anxious about what they are doing, some of course are more cautious about judicial intervention than others, and some are troubled by the prospect of issuing a judicial order which they know the state will disobey. They recognize that these cases drag on for decades. But one thing is clear: once a litigating attorney succeeds in getting a judge to visit a public mental institution, there is a very good chance that that judge will conclude that something has to be done, and that the Constitution gives him or her the power to do it. The Justices of the Supreme Court, however, cannot be made to visit the children's facilities in Georgia, the state mental hospitals in Alabama, the institutions for the mentally retarded in Pennsylvania. The ultimate decision makers decide the rule of law at a remove from reality.

At the beginning of this essay I set out the three major policy questions: the power of psychiatry, the autonomy of the patient, and the paternalistic obligations of the state. The Supreme Court has in its own convoluted way reasserted the power of the psychiatrist. The Justices have done this despite the protestations of civil libertarians and even against the wishes of the American Psychiatric Association. They have insisted that psychiatrists have the power to predict dangerousness in the courtroom. (But this empowering of psychiatrists is meaningless as I shall demonstrate in the next chapter.) They have paid lip service to the autonomy of the patient, but none of their decisions has strengthened the patient's right to be left alone. As to forcing the states to meet the needs of patients, they have done the least that was possible. The only coherent policy that seems to have been served is minimal judicial activism. At least that is how it looks to me as, like Kafka's peasant, I wait at my door to the law.

REFERENCES

1. *Parham v. J. R.*, 442 U.S. 584, 624–625 (1979).

2. 345 N.Y.S.2d 560, 42 A.D.2d 559 (N.Y. App. Div. 1973), *aff'd* 33 N.Y.2d 902, 352 N.Y.S.2d 626 (N.Y. 1973), *cert. dismissed* 420 U.S. 307 (1975).

3. 339 U.S. 9 (1950).

4. *Ibid.*, p. 23.

5. *Ibid.*, p. 23.

6. 406 U.S. 715 (1972).

7. *Ibid.*, p. 737.

8. *Ibid.*, p. 737.

9. 408 U.S. 238 (1972).

10. Tex. Crim. Proc. Code Ann. Sec 37.071 (B)(2)(Vern), 1981.

11. American Bar Association, *Criminal Justice Mental Health Standards* (First Tentative Draft), July 1983.

12. *Jurek v. Texas*, 428 U.S. 262 (1976).

13. *Ibid.*, pp. 275–276.

14. 451 U.S. 454 (1981).

15. *Ibid.*, p. 454, n. 8 ("The American Psychiatric Association suggests . . . that absent a defendant's willingness to cooperate . . . a psychiatric examination would be meaningless [for predicting future dangerousness]. *Brief* for American Psychiatric Association as *Amicus Curiae* at 26.")

16. *Estelle*, 451 U.S. at 472.

17. *Barefoot v. State*, 596 S.W.2d 875 (Tex. Crim. App. 1980).

18. *Barefoot*, 697 F.2d at 596 (5th Cir. 1983).

19. *Ibid.*, p. 596.

20. *Barefoot*, 453 U.S. 913.

21. *O'Connor v. Donaldson*, 422 U.S. 563 (1975).

22. B. Woodward and S. Armstrong, *The Brethren* (Simon and Schuster, 1979), p. 372.

23. T. Szasz, *Psychiatric Slavery* (Free Press, 1977), p. 15; and B. Ennis, *Prisoners of Psychiatry* (Harcourt, Brace, Jovanovich, 1972), p. 84.

24. T. Szasz, *op. cit.*, pp. 14, 17.

25. *Donaldson v. O'Connor*, 493 F.2d 507, 510 (5th Cir. 1974).

26. *Ibid.*, p. 511.

27. 42 U.S.C. §1983 (1979).

28. 325 F.Supp. 781 (M.D. Ala. 1971), *on submission of proposed standards by defendants,* 334 F.Supp. 1341 (M.D. Ala. 1971), *enforced* 344 F.Supp. 373 (M.D. Ala. 1972).

29. *Donaldson v. O'Connor,* 493 F.2d 507 (5th Cir. 1974).

30. *Wyatt v. Aderholt,* 503 F.2d 1305 (5th Cir. 1974).

31. *Donaldson,* 493 F.2d at 520.

32. B. Woodward and S. Armstrong, *op. cit.,* p. 372.

33. *O'Connor.* 422 U.S. at 578 (Burger, C. J., concurring).

34. *Ibid.*, p. 577, n. 12.

35. *Ibid.*, p. 587–588.

36. *Addington v. Texas,* 441 U.S. 418 (1979).

37. *Application of Gault,* 387 U.S. 1 (1967).

38. *Parham,* 442 U.S. 609.

39. *Ibid.*, p. 609.

40. *Jones v. United States,* 103 S.Ct. 3043 (1983).

41. *Halderman v. Pennhurst State School and Hospital,* 446 F.Supp. 1295 (E.D. Pa. 1978).

42. *Halderman v. Pennhurst State School and Hospital,* 612 F.2d 84 (3rd Cir. 1982) *(en banc).*

43. 42 U.S.C. §§6001 *et seq.* (1976 ed. and Supp.III).

44. 42 U.S.C. §§6010(1) & (2).

45. *Pennhurst State School and Hospital v. Halderman,* 451 U.S. 1, 18 (1981).

46. *Ibid.*, p. 19.

47. *Halderman v. Pennhurst State School and Hospital,* 673 F.2d 647, 665 (3rd Cir. 1982)(Garth, J., concurring in part and dissenting as to relief).

48. *Cert. granted, Pennhurst State School and Hospital v. Halderman,* 457 U.S. 1131 (1982).

49. 707 F.2d 702 (3rd Cir. 1983).

50. *Ibid.*, p. 706.

51. *Ibid.*, p. 707.

52. *Ibid.*, p. 709.

53. *Ibid.*, p. 715.

54. *Romeo v. Youngberg*, 102 S.Ct. 2452 (1982).

55. *Romeo v. Youngberg*, 644 F.2d 147 (3rd Cir. 1980).

56. *Ibid.*, p. 164.

57. *Ibid.*, p. 169.

58. *Romeo v. Youngberg, op. cit.*, 102 S.Ct. at 2458.

59. *Ibid.*, p. 2459.

60. *Ibid.*, p. 2458, n. 20.

61. *Ibid.*, p. 2463 (Blackmun, J., concurring).

62. *Ibid.*, p. 2465 (Burger, C. J., concurring).

VI

Psychiatric Abuse and Legal Reform: Two Ways to Make a Bad Situation Worse

JUSTICE POTTER STEWART writing in *Parham v. J.R.* expressed a point of view which as I suggested in the previous chapter seems to me crucial for those of us who are seriously concerned about the troubling intersections between law and psychiatry. "Issues concerning mental illness are among the most difficult that courts have to face, involving as they often do serious problems of policy disguised as questions of constitutional law."[1]

I have taken Justice Stewart's words as comfort for my own opinion that there are very few sacred or lapidary constitutional answers in our difficult field. It would seem that policy considerations properly include psychiatric views about mental illness, treatment, social costs, and benefits. It would also seem that criticism of new constitutional claims cannot be dismissed by a string of citations and the bald assertion that the unfortunate consequences of a court's constitutional ruling are irrelevant.

If Justice Stewart is correct about our field, as I believe he is, imagine the extraordinary difficulties a judge confronts in making mental health policy. Not only is the discipline itself filled with controversy, conflict, and uncertainty,[2] it is also a subject about which all of us, judges included, are apt to have charged feelings as a result of some personal or family experience. A further handicap to dealing with these serious problems of policy is that courts must resolve the issues before them, issues which typically get narrower and narrower as they move up the appellate ladder. This narrowing of issues makes cases more decidable, but it also wrenches them out of their social context and reality, so that the court often must struggle with broad policy problems while exercising judicial tunnel vision. The *Parham* case itself as I demonstrated was a most striking example of this process. The lower court's decision[3] had adopted as policy the recommendations of a commission which had evaluated Georgia's inpatient services for children and found them wanting. The three-judge court in essence copied the recommendations of the commission into its decision. It made no effort to disguise the serious policy problems as constitutional issues. That happened only in the Supreme Court, where the question of the quality of institutions for children fell outside the court's tunnel vision, as it narrowed the issue to consider only the rights of parents and the constitutional requirements of due process for the admission of children to mental health facilities.

As I pointed out in the last chapter, the Supreme Court dealt with *O'Connor v. Donaldson*[4] and *Addington v. Texas*[5] in much the same way, narrowing its focus so as to avoid the serious policy problems that arose from the lower federal courts. It has done the same with the right to refuse treatment and has done as little as possible with the right to habilitation. The court seems particularly unwilling to do anything in the law and psychiatry area which will cost money. In *Schweiker v. Wilson*,[6] for example, the Court refused to award to mental patients from ages twenty-one to sixty-four in public institutions the twenty-five dollars per month allowance for sundry personal expenses that other disabled institutionalized persons receive under Medicaid.

The lower federal courts that have issued the benchmark decisions on involuntary confinement and treatment have had a somewhat broader perspective.[7] They have taken on more, and they have been quite willing to force the states to expend large amounts. But in their legal policies which have resulted in the "criminalization" of the mental health system, they have, I think, demonstrated the limitations of the legal imagination. Imposing the standards and procedures of the criminal law (criminalization) may give judges a comforting sense of uniformity and familiarity, but that does not mean it is a wise or prudent or rational method of selecting patients for admission to hospitals. However, much of the legal reform in mental health law has come not from judges but from legislatures which presumably are free to canvass every aspect of policy before they vote to change a law. Most states have rewritten their mental health laws and all have moved in the direction of criminalization, the underlying premise of which is that the only valid justification for confinement is that the person poses an imminent threat to society. The states have all retained other substantive criteria, such as danger to self and "gravely disabled," but the central thrust of reform is to make danger to society rather than need for treatment the basic legal policy of civil commitment.[8] This is the direction urged by the American Civil Liberties Union, by the Mental Health Law Project, by the Justice Department, by many legal scholars, and by a variety of other groups concerned about individual autonomy and the excessive powers of psychiatry. The most extraordinary psychological paradox of these years of legal ferment and change is that the reformers saw psychiatrists as persons of enormous power who had to be restrained by law, and the psychiatrists saw themselves as powerless from the start and helpless by the end. At any rate, I shall argue that criminalization, whenever adopted by legislators or imposed by judges, is bad policy. I believe that legislatures adopted it because it was packaged and presented as part of the civil rights movement, a substantial civil libertarian reform that could be accomplished with beneficial fiscal consequences.[9] And I believe civil libertarians pushed for these reforms without sufficiently being concerned about the disabling impact of serious mental disorders.

As the title of this essay suggests, I intend to discuss psychiatric abuse as well as mistaken legal reforms. No doubt I have overstated my case in what follows, but I believe that so much radical change has occurred at the juncture between law and psychiatry that it is time for both sides to look back very critically and ask what have we done wrong. I hope that addressing that question will tell us something about where we go from here.

Although the term "psychiatric abuse" implies a knowing or intentional action by a single actor, abuse can be both unknowing and unintended. I shall use the term to include also failures of collective responsibility which, in the aggregate, cause harm. Indeed, even psychiatric *reform* can make a bad situation worse and result in abuse.

With these considerations in mind, I present the following bill of particulars, some of which I have already touched on in these essays.

(1) Psychiatric and legal reform have together increased the risk of violence to the public by the dangerously mentally ill. Criminalization has failed to do the one legitimate thing it was supposed to do—protect the public.

(2) The greatest failing of the modern mental health system, causing the most suffering to patients, has been the failure of continuity of care. Legal reform has intensified this problem at every turn.

(3) The greatest professional ethical failing of modern psychiatry, and indeed all of medicine, has been the abandonment of the responsibility that runs to the patient as a person. Instead, the doctor defines his role in some narrower technical sense. Legal reform has made it easier for psychiatrists to justify and rationalize this failure of responsibility.

(4) The psychiatric profession has consistently, over the years, found ways to avoid caring for the sickest patients. Legal reform has, if anything, increased this trend.

(5) The psychiatric profession has never adequately staffed public mental hospitals, which disproportionately serve the poor and minorities. Legal reform has driven still more qualified psychiatrists out of the public sector.

(6) Psychiatry has traditionally done a bad job with families, blaming them and making them feel guilty. Legal reform has alienated the family and in that process has made the natural caretakers of the mentally ill, and their families, helpless in the face of crisis and suffering.

(7) In the past, some of the worst abuses in psychiatry resulted when psychiatrists acted as policemen rather than as therapists. Legal reform has consistently undermined the therapeutic role and forced the psychiatrist into the role of policeman.

(8) The inappropriate prescribing of tranquilizers has been one of the great scandals of medicine in general, and of psychiatry in particular. Legal reform, by singling out for regulation and control what the courts call antipsychotic drugs, has created new incentives for inappropriate drug treatment and has made less accessible what for many patients is the single most effective treatment available.

Obviously, an enormous amount of empirical evidence is necessary to document all these claims. I do not have that evidence. But as President of the American Psychiatric Association and first Chair of its Commission on Judicial Action I have been at the center of the psychiatric profession and in the middle of many of the legal developments of the past decade, and I shall draw on that experience. Again, my hope is to provoke both psychiatrists and lawyers to stop to reflect about what we have done wrong.

I shall discuss the eight items in my bill of particulars under four headings. First I shall consider the risks of violence; second, continuity, responsibility, and treatment of the sickest patients; and third, alienation of the family. Finally, using the recent cases on the right to refuse treatment as a context, I shall consider the psychiatrist as policeman and the abuses of drugs.

THE RISKS OF VIOLENCE

The general public, I think, would expect an essay with the title I have given this one to describe how psychiatrists who have no sense of morality and lawyers who care nothing about victims have undermined law and order and left the public at the mercy of dangerous madmen. The murder of John Lennon and the attempted assassination of President Reagan (see Chapter IV) are only the most glaring examples of what the mass media vividly present as senseless violence committed by deranged people who should have been confined, or, even worse, by deranged people who have been released from confinement.[10] Violence is frightening enough, but senseless violence and violence that could have been prevented are horrifying, and it gives special intensity to the growing public concern that society has somehow lost an important measure of necessary protection.

Is the public right? Are they less protected? Have psychiatrists and lawyers tilted the scales against public protection?

As I mentioned in the essay on Psychiatry and Violence, there are three interrelated legal systems for controlling identified violent adults: the criminal justice system; the quasi-criminal justice system, which includes all those legal procedures for confining mentally ill offenders; and the mental health system. During the past few years as a spokesman for the American psychiatric establishment, I have learned that journalists, talk show hosts, the educated citizenry, and even some distinguished members of the legal profession believe that psychiatry has somehow corrupted the criminal justice system. The claims are sometimes inarticulate, but the conviction is passionate and growing. A recurrent element in these claims is that psychiatric ideas have somehow muddied the moral and behavioral premises that run through the criminal law. The most obvious specific example of this loss of conceptual clarity is the notion of diminished capacity, or more generally the admission of psychiatric testimony on the issue of *mens rea* (criminal intent) as well as in support of the insanity defense. I believe that these objections have some validity but are trivial when seen in proper perspective. As I pointed out in the chapter on Psychiatry and

Violence, when the vast majority of criminal cases are disposed of by plea bargaining,[11] when first offenders convicted of armed robbery are routinely given suspended sentences,[12] when one arrest in a hundred ends in a prison sentence,[13] when the fate of criminals depends on the quality of their lawyers, then the muddying of *mens rea* is not the problem. If the criminal justice system has lost some of its ability to deter violence, to protect society, and to exact retribution, then it needs to look beyond psychiatry.

Now what of the quasi-criminal justice system: incompetency, the insanity defense, statutes allowing for special confinement of the sexually dangerous or the defective delinquent? The psychiatrist plays a major role in this system, and the public is particularly concerned about the insanity defense as an important and dangerous exception to the rule of law. Once again, of course, when seen in perspective, these are relatively rare events, but because the insanity defense is often invoked in the most publicized trials one can understand why it looms so large in the public imagination.[14] (Paradoxically, some of the most publicized cases of recent years have not raised the insanity defense. For example, the trial of Sirhan Sirhan and Dan White's "Twinkie Defense" involved California's defense of diminished capacity. Son of Sam and Mark David Chapman, who killed John Lennon, both pleaded guilty.)

And it is in the quasi-criminal area that considerable legal reform has occurred which has not been fully appreciated by the public. *Jackson v. Indiana*,[15] as we saw, signaled the end of lifetime confinement as the penalty for being incompetent to stand trial. Similarly, giving new due process safeguards to sexual psychopaths,[16] requiring commitment hearings before confinement of those found not guilty by reason of insanity,[17] and equally important statutory reforms governing the locus of confinement[18] have made it more difficult to lock up the dangerous mentally ill, and periodic review has made it more difficult to keep them locked up. At every point where the criminal justice system in fact relied on the mental health system for an extra measure of public security, that extra measure has been found legally suspect. I do not intend to question the "rightness" or the "constitutional necessity" of these reforms, but I think it is important to acknowledge the costs which some reformers have ignored. "Incompetent" and "not guilty by reason of insanity" no longer constitute easy judicial and prosecutorial dispositions guaranteeing long hospital stays in high security institutions. Steadman's remarkable study on the outcome of being found not guilty by reason of insanity in New York makes that clear.[19] Recidivism by the criminally insane is now an important issue of public concern.

Nor can the criminal courts obtain the public security they once achieved by ordinary civil commitment—the third system for controlling violent persons. New substantive criteria, due process safeguards, and periodic review make that impossible. It is important to realize that the reforms of the second and third systems took place when the criminal justice system was already in advanced congestive failure and could not take up new burdens.

Professor Alan Dershowitz likes to talk about confinement as a balloon: squeeze it here, it sticks out there.[20] The idea is that society will confine a certain number and kind of people, if not in mental institutions, then in penal institutions. But there can be no doubt that in this country during the past decade a great deal of air has been let out of the balloon.[21] Many of those released were harmless people improperly confined in terrible institutions, but a few were dangerously mentally ill persons. Their freedom is the price society pays for reform and its new due process safeguards, a price they have now begun to realize.

Law makers, of course, have tried to control that price. The basic policy argument in all of this constitutional litigation and statutory reform has been two-pronged. First, the only moral justification for confining persons not convicted of crimes is that they pose a threat to society; the crucial substantive criterion is thus dangerousness.[22] The second prong of the argument is that if we stop wasting our resources on the harmless, we can more effectively deal with those who are violent. Whether or not the first prong of the argument is morally correct, by now it is clear that the second prong, the expectation of greater effectiveness in dealing with violent patients, was incorrect.

In 1973 the president of the National Council of Crime and Delinquency wrote that the identification of dangerous persons was "the greatest unresolved problem the criminal justice system faces."[23] Yet every court and legislature that has revised its mental health laws has made this "unresolved problem" in criminal justice the key to reforming the mental health system. A finding of dangerousness now determines whether a person will be confined after being found incompetent to stand trial[24] or not guilty by reason of insanity.[25] Similarly, such findings determine who is civilly committed[26] and who is sentenced to death in some states.[27]

I need not present here the difficulties inherent in determining dangerousness. They are well known. In response to this civil commitment problem, some civil libertarians have proposed a past act requirement.[28] But the past act requirement does not eliminate the prediction problem. The past act standard gives the dog one bite, then postpones prediction until a decision has to be made about discharge. Even if mental health practitioners were capable of making the short-term predictions Professor Monahan hopes they can make,[29] such predictions do not apply to discharge decisions, for reasons Professor Halleck long ago made clear.[30]

Thus far, I mean to suggest that, to the extent that judges and legislatures believed that these legal reforms embodied a policy which did not sacrifice the public safety, they were wrong, and they may have misled the public as well.

The law must rest on a morally sound foundation, but for the system of law to function at all, the moral premise must be able to generate clear and concrete empirical distinctions. If it cannot, then the law in practice becomes irrational and incoherent. I believe that the concept of dangerousness does not generate clear, concrete empirical distinctions. When the Supreme Court acknowledges that it is difficult to decide who is dangerous, but tells courts to make such decisions anyway, it embraces incoherence.[31]

But to stop here would be to paint a grossly misleading and unfair picture, for this story has another side—how psychiatry has contributed to the loss of public protection. Until the second half of this century, long-term custodial confinement was an accepted practice of institutional psychiatry.[32] Whether patients were dangerous or not and whether they came from the criminal courts by quasi-criminal procedures or by ordinary civil commitment, the length of hospital stay could often be measured in years rather than days. "Twenty five years ago the average length of hospitalization in the United States for schizophrenia was 13.1 years."[33] As long as psychiatry endorsed or accepted the practice of long-term custodial confinement, mental institutions provided an extra measure of protection for the criminal justice system. Psychiatry, by calling custodial confinement "treatment," gave legitimacy to the practice of locking people up for the rest of their lives whether they were dangerous or not.

Later, when the community mental health system approach began to dominate the therapeutic imagination and psychiatrists opened their eyes to the evils of long-term institutionalization, a process began which even without legal reform might well have ended many of the abuses the civil libertarians decried. But these changes also radically altered the mental health system's ability to protect society. Institutions with revolving doors offer little security to the public. When therapeutic considerations alone determine the length of hospital stay, patients who would formerly have been hospitalized for months or years are now often released after only a few days. By 1971 the median length of hospital stay in state and county mental hospitals, which presumably serve the sickest patients, was forty-one days. During the decade of the 1980s we can expect the median to be three weeks.[34] Inevitably, then, the public security objective conflicts with therapeutic objectives, most dramatically in the cases of those found not guilty by reason of insanity. The vast majority of people who are psychotic when they kill someone will have had all of the hospital treatment they require before their trial is held. If they are to be confined in hospitals after the trial at which they are found not guilty by reason of insanity, it will not be for compelling therapeutic reasons. Again, the dominant therapeutic ideology no longer serves public security nor will it legitimize lifetime confinement as treatment.

The criminal justice system can no longer enjoy the luxury of hypocrisy. Courts can no longer find someone not guilty by reason of insanity and then declare that they are not punishing him when they lock him up for the rest of his life. Perhaps for the first time in its history the insanity defense has bite.

This analysis is of course as oversimplified as was my analysis of legal developments, but my purpose here is to stand back and look from a distance at the broad outlines. Looking back from the 1980s we can see that psychiatrists and civil libertarians have been heading in the same general direction.

CONTINUITY OF CARE, RESPONSIBILITY FOR PATIENTS, AND TREATMENT OF THE SICKEST PATIENTS

John J. Paris, after a clear critical damning analysis of the New York court's early right-to-die decisions,[35] urged the medical profession to ignore the courts and continue to do what is right. I think Paris should have directed his plea to the lawyers who advise the hospitals where people go to die. Their job is to keep the hospital free from legal risk, or at least to minimize those risks. What would those lawyers do if the medical staff met and voted to follow Paris' advice? Is it not more likely that those hospital lawyers are already drafting regulations to comply with the courts' decision and that the hospital staff will go along?

One of the unfortunate consequences of the increase in malpractice liability is the phenomenon of defensive medicine. Doctors concerned about their own civil liability, with or without the advice of lawyers, impose on patients unnecessary tests and procedures which not only add to the growing cost of health care but expose the patient to un-necessary risks. Typically the doctor and his lawyer have an exaggerated sense of legal liability and an insufficient appreciation of the aggregate risks to patients. Defensive medicine is, of course, an unintended consequence of law, but every new malpractice decision is in some sense a new regulation of the practice of medicine. Similarly, every reform of mental health law and every mental health decision of the Federal Courts under the civil rights provisions of the United States Code (Title 42, Section 1983) has a regulatory effect on the practice of psychiatry, particularly practice in the public sector. Section 1983 allows suits for alleged violations of civil rights. Most mental health cases have come under this rubric, a few have actually sought monetary damages. Since each Department of Mental Health, like every large general hospital, by now has its own legal bureaucracy spinning out regulations, many doctors are simply overwhelmed. I had the impression during the course of the *Rogers v. Okin* trial, a Section 1983 suit concerning the right to refuse treatment, that the doctors simply did not know or comprehend their state's own regulations on seclusion,[36] which seemed to have been drafted by lawyers from the American Civil Liberties Union without regard for clinical realities or accepted practice. Many doctors are genuinely confused about what they can and cannot do.[37] There is a pervasive conviction in public mental hospitals that the law has made it impossible to treat people who don't want treatment, so why bother. Being a psychiatrist seems to require acts of civil disobedi-ence which few are willing to perform. Instead, psychiatrists merely go through the motions without feeling responsible. A typical reaction is for psychiatrists to assume that patients cannot be involuntarily con-fined; perhaps in identification with the aggressor, they make not a clinical judgment but a legal judgment. They interpret the law in a very strict and limited fashion, as though they were prosecutors who wanted to win all their cases. Whatever their motives, the bottom line is this: I am helpless to do anything because of the law and I am not responsible.

Recently I was asked to consult on a patient who was being held on temporary commitment in a community mental health center. The patient had had over twenty such temporary commitments, though he was not yet twenty-three years old. Each hospitalization was precipi-tated by some minor act of public violence; this last time he had pushed his priest. Throughout this whole series of hospitalizations, there had never been a sustained effort to treat this patient, who was uncoopera-tive and frightening to the staff. None of the mental health practitioners understood or had a relationship with him, nor did any of them really have an interest in him or any idea how to treat him. When I interviewed the man, he was clearly not psychotic, nor was there any evidence that he ever had been. He had been evaluated neurologically and the findings were negative. He was of rather low intelligence, had never finished grammar school, and had no job skills. The chief finding of my mental-status exam was that he smelled of liquor and seemed to be drunk. Since the mental health center was in the middle of the city and not very secure, this was certainly not impossible. Here was a patient selected for hospitalization not by medical criteria but by the criteria of the criminalized civil commitment statute. Hospitalization as treatment was a charade. The psychiatric staff was merely observing the legal niceties; certainly this revolving-door facility was not secure and confinement had no value as treatment or as public protection.

This patient's case contrasts sharply with that of another young man, who was the subject of the Massachusetts Supreme Court's landmark decision dealing with the right to refuse treatment.[38] Richard Roe III, after an apparently untroubled childhood that was marked by success and apparent popularity in school, began at sixteen years of age to become withdrawn and seclusive. His academic performance deteriorated, and he was seriously involved with alcohol, marijuana, and LSD. He was eventually expelled from the private school he attended and enrolled in public school, but did poorly and dropped out without graduating. While in high school, he was evaluated under the provisions of the Massachusetts law which provides for assessment of and appropriate education for disabled children.[39] The evaluation resulted in a recommendation that Richard Roe be admitted to a psychiatric hospital.

This young man was on a classic downhill course. But he was not actually committed for psychiatric observation until after criminal charges of receiving stolen property were brought against him. The psychiatrists diagnosed him as schizophrenic, and having done their "legal" task he was discharged to his fate in the criminal justice system, which typically did nothing. The referral for diagnostic evaluation had been the court's disposition of the case. In the hospital he had refused both medication and other treatment. Returned to his home, he exhibited bizarre behavior, "wearing a fur coat for hours on extremely hot days and standing for prolonged periods of time with a water glass poised at his lips."[40] His family repeatedly tried to induce him to seek help, but he refused any kind of treatment. Six months after his first hospitalization he was again committed for observation after being charged with attempted unarmed robbery and assault and battery. While hospitalized he attacked another patient for no apparent reason. He again refused antipsychotic medication and refused to participate in psychotherapy. Again the hospital apparently just gave up and made plans to discharge him to his fate in the criminal justice system. His father, following what were then the requirements of *Rogers v. Okin*,[41] sought appointment as guardian to impose the drug treatment his son refused.

At the hearing, there was considerable ambiguity about the son's reasons for refusing medication. Supposedly his experience with illicit drugs had caused him an automobile accident, and on that basis he was opposed to licit drugs. On the other hand, a lawyer acting as his guardian *ad litem*, and contesting his father's appointment as guardian and the delegation of drug decisions, claimed that the young man had accepted certain tenets of the Christian Science Church, and refused drugs for that reason. The testimony at the initial hearing established to a judge's satisfaction that the young man was seriously mentally ill, that his judgment was gravely impaired, that he needed treatment, and that he could not make informed decisions. The judge did not believe he was a Christian Scientist. But Richard Roe III apparently never got treated.

At a second hearing on permanent guardianship, three psychiatrists were called to testify. All agreed that the young man was mentally ill. Two psychiatrists said he was schizophrenic, that his judgment was seriously impaired, and that he exhibited a pattern of intense, abrupt anger. The psychiatrist called by the guardian *ad litem* testified that the patient was competent to care for himself in a limited sense. He acknowledged that the patient was incapable of carrying on a reasonable conversation, was unable to live in a community by himself, was deteriorating, and could not participate in interpersonal social situations without impulsive rage reactions. The court appointed the father guardian, but ordered that he not be allowed to impose antipsychotic drug treatment on the son until the question of his right to refuse treatment was decided by the Massachusetts Supreme Judicial Court.

Both of these cases illustrate the ludicrous waste of human resources and public funds which the present system, with its tragicomic mixture of psychiatric abuse and legal reform, encourages. In the first case, mechanical application of criminalized standards results in a young man being endlessly and expensively sent to hospitals; he only ends up stigmatized as crazy, receiving no help for his other obvious limitations. He certainly receives no meaningful treatment, nor is it clear that any is available. It is often this kind of patient who now costs society the greatest expense. Not really a criminal and not having a treatable mental illness, he moves in and out of the mental health and the criminal justice systems. A report of a similar case indicated that the patient-defendant, in a few years, had cost over a quarter of a million dollars in public funds due to arrests, bookings, and psychiatric evaluations alone.[42] In the second case, three psychiatrists and two judges agree that a young man is psychotic, yet he apparently can gain admission to a mental hospital only by being charged with a crime. He is sinking into schizophrenia and there is a good chance he can be treated, yet—at enormous legal expense to his family and the taxpayers—the law is seeing to it that his autonomy is preserved and that he will not get timely or appropriate treatment. Whatever policies the legislatures and courts may have intended to further, it is clear in these cases, which are not atypical, that reform has made a bad situation worse.

Legal writers have repeatedly noted that psychiatrists, when challenged about civil commitment or told there will be a full hearing on a case, will change their minds and back off.[43] This tendency is often cited as evidence of the arbitrariness or unreliability of psychiatric diagnoses and decision-making, but that, it seems to me, is an unfortunate misinterpretation. On the one hand it reflects those psychiatrists' lack of any serious sense of responsibility for the patient. On the other hand, the psychiatrist has neither the training nor the temperament to be a prosecutor. The psychiatrist regards civil commitment as an unpleasant duty, not as a personal responsibility. If the psychiatrist finds it becoming more unpleasant, he gives it up. The vast majority of psychiatrists are not interested in matching wits with a lawyer. Indeed the growing problem in many states as mentioned is that psychiatrists assume that the law is against *them* and they are therefore reluctant to commit anyone. Not only does this reluctance affect the psychiatrist involved in legal proceedings, it also has an important impact on psychiatric decision-makers dealing with patients in other contexts. The psychiatrist who knows that he will have difficulty managing a problem patient and that legal constraints will make him unable to control the course of treatment will conclude that he is not personally responsible for the outcome.

Even without legal reform, the single most important and harmful practice in the mental health system during the past decade has been the failure to provide continuity of care.[44] Legal activists with their eyes firmly fastened on the past may have contributed to this abuse, but they did not invent it. The community mental health approach offered psychiatry a conceptual rationale for short-term treatment. But the most dominant force in the structure of modern medicine, third-party payment, offers the most powerful of all professional incentives for short-term treatment—money. Psychiatry began to change from a specialty with a low turnover of patients who were seen for a long time to one with a high turnover of patients seen for a short time. This trend appeared not only in community mental health centers and state hospitals with revolving-door policies, and in profitable new private psychiatric hospitals and the new psychiatric wards of general hospitals, but also in the offices of increasing numbers of private practitioners. Powerful psychotropic drugs, crisis-oriented treatment, short-term therapies, whatever their value as treatment, also had an economic virtue. If third-party payment paid for ten office visits, it was convenient to have a treatment method that took only ten office visits. If third-party payment paid only for brief hospital stays, then it was fortunate that one could get a patient in, medicate him, deal with the crisis quickly, and get him out. The American infatuation with long-term therapy was coming to an end. The entire profession of medicine was going through its own spontaneous explosion of technical, diagnostic, and treatment procedures. And this, too, was being enhanced by the structure of third-party payment, which rewarded the doctor for the number and complexity of his procedures rather than for the quality and continuity of care provided his patients.[45]

Psychiatry could not keep pace with the technically and financially rewarding ingenuity of other specialties. It gradually sank in comparative income to near the bottom of the specialist ladder.[46] This decline created still more incentive for high volume, short-term treatment. In this therapeutic atmosphere the sickest patients are given drugs, often without adequate psychiatric supervision, with no attempt at a therapeutic alliance and with no sense of individual responsibility. Indeed in many mental health centers the patient is treated by nonpsychiatrists and the psychiatrist has been reduced to signing prescriptions for "patients" who are other people's "clients." This in my view is institutionalizing malpractice. There are of course responsible psychiatrists giving good care to very sick patients, but the sickest patients are often uncooperative and legal reform has put obstacles in the way of responsible care.

There can be no question that economic incentives, together with the new therapeutic rationales, moved the psychiatric practitioner and psychiatric institutions away from continuity of care. Legal reform has added to this pressure. Indeed, it has allowed mental health practitioners to rationalize a growing and pervasive sense that since they cannot have authority they need not feel a personal responsibility for very sick patients. And this is not all rationalization; the psychiatrist's hands have been tied by new statutes, new constitutional holdings, and a rhetoric of rights which issues in a mass of regulations.[47]

DEFECTION FROM THE PUBLIC SECTOR

For more than thirty years American psychiatry has publicly recognized its failure to recruit enough qualified psychiatrists for public mental hospitals. The void has been partially filled by foreign medical gradu-ates,[48] many of whom are not licensed to practice anywhere else. But there have always been a certain number of do-gooders—qualified psychiatrists who, whether trained here or abroad, make their career in the public sector and by their own example of service recruit a few others. I cannot tell you how many of these good psychiatrists have given up on practice in the public sector, and not just for economic reasons. They feel they have been rendered impotent, and, I think equally important, they feel unappreciated.

There is a psychological reality here which ought not to be too difficult for lawyers to grasp. Imagine a lawyer who has gone to work in an inner city legal aid office and has undertaken to provide a range of le-gal services. If she does her work well, it will consume all her energies while compensating her much less well than does the corporate work her classmates have chosen. Her work is a cause which claims her convictions and her dedication—she is a do-gooder. Suddenly there appears on the scene a regime which polemically asserts that she has been abusing her clients, misrepresenting their legal needs to fulfill her own ideology, and making unnecessary use of intrusive legal methods with dangerous side effects, such as the class action suit, which highly qualified legal experts claim has totally unpredictable long-term side effects. And she is told that all available openings for lawyers in the legal aid office will be filled by paralegals who are fully qualified to do what lawyers do, cost less, and are more available. If the analogy is to be complete, then the legal aid office must retain and pay from its limited funds a team of psychiatrists to advise on any case that has possible psychological implications. Intrusive methods like the class action suit must first be approved by a committee of psychiatrists who will decide whether the named plaintiffs have in fact been given all of the legal information they need to make an informed decision. The psychiatrists will also fully explore the legal issues and must be convinced that no less drastic alternative is available.

If one can imagine what it would be like to practice law under those constraints, one can begin to understand what it is like to practice psychiatry in the public sector in the decade of the 1980s. Since I have engaged in a flight of fancy to suggest the psychological realities, let me quote Judge Aldisert dissenting in *Romeo v. Youngberg*[49] (discussed in Psychiatry and the Supreme Court, Chapter 5) to show that this is something more than an exercise in autistic thinking by a psychiatrist. Various members of the staff of an institution for the mentally retarded had been sued for damages for violating the constitutional rights of patients. Commenting on the incredibly complicated constitutional regulations for liability which the majority had fashioned, Aldisert gave the following advice: "If you are contemplating a position as an attendant in a mental hospital, seek another job! There is simply too much unpredictability in the law governing your conduct. If you are a physician, make certain that the state's malpractice insurance policy includes a clause protecting you from the new 'constitutional torts' manufactured today by the Third Circuit Court of Appeals."[50]

Judge Aldisert does not give adequate attention to the ambiguities of malpractice liability insurance and its applicability to damages arising out of a lawsuit claiming deprivation of civil rights rather than medical negligence. Nor does he take into account all of the other legal regulations of the public sector. If he were to do so, he might give physicians the same advice he gives attendants.

Obviously there are other considerations beside legal regulation that have led to defection from the public sector. The displacement of psychiatrists by other mental health professions as well as the other economic, professional, and personal inducements are also important. But my point is that legal regulation has not helped and it is certainly often given as a reason by psychiatrists for leaving the public sector.

ALIENATION OF THE FAMILY

The fate of most people with serious mental illness is to be abandoned by their families, as Hollingshead and Redlich[51] demonstrated twenty-five years ago and as every experienced clinician can confirm from experience. Psychiatrists facilitated this abandonment by confining patients in distant mental hospitals and by making families feel guilty and inadequate. The development of a family-oriented psychiatry, the recognition of the problem of the identified patient,[52] and other developments to involve the family rather than exclude them were important corrective measures. But families with a seriously disabled member need help; living with a psychotic person can be devastating. An enlightened policy would ensure that families are supported and encouraged to keep mentally disabled persons at home, but it would facilitate treatment, recognizing that without help the pressure to abandon or exclude the mentally ill person only increases. The most dramatic example of legal reform that runs directly counter to such policy occurred in *Bartley v. Kremens*.[53] Enlightened programs for mentally retarded children include a respite program. Families are allowed to place their retarded child in some appropriate facility for a week or two so that they can have a respite from the extraordinary burden of caring for such a child. Yet the lower federal court in *Bartley* concluded that such a case presents a constitutional conflict of interest between parents and child, and that the child should have a lawyer, a legal hearing, and the opportunity to contest the respite practice.[54]

The assumption of a conflict of interest between the family and the patient articulated by the lower court in *Bartley*[55] has become the basic assumption in legal reform of mental health law. The case of Richard Roe III, whom I have already mentioned, is another dramatic example. He presented the legal problem of the right to refuse treatment of a mentally ill patient outside the mental hospital. The Supreme Court of Massachusetts accepted the finding that he was schizophrenic and deteriorating, they found him incompetent, they agreed that his father should be appointed his permanent guardian, but they concluded that in the absence of an emergency as defined by Webster's dictionary, his father could not impose on him the "antipsychotic drugs" urged by the psychiatrist. "We think that the possibility that the ward's schizophrenia might deteriorate into a chronic, irreversible condition at an uncertain but relatively distant date does not satisfy our definition of emergency."[56]

The courts face two central questions in consent cases involving incompetents. First, who should make treatment decisions for the incompetent: the next of kin, a guardian *ad litem*, a judge, a patients' rights committee, or the attending physicians? As we saw in *Bartley* the civil libertarian view in the psychiatric context disfavors the family or next of kin and favors due process and a judge. Second, what standard should the substitute decision-maker use in deciding what treatment to authorize? Most commonly, courts instruct the decision-maker to act "in the best interests of the patient."[57] But this standard itself gives little real guidance; the decision-maker is left to choose whether to respect what he supposes to be the incompetent's actual wishes,[58] or to do what a "reasonable person" would do in the incompetent's position,

or simply to follow the recommendations of the doctors.[59] Massachusetts decided in *Roe* and later in *Rogers v. Commissioner of Mental
Health*[60] to attempt to act on the preferences of the particular incompetent patient.

The court has ruled that judges in making substituted judgments
should consider six factors: (1) the patient's expressed preferences;
(2) the patient's religious convictions; (3) the interest of the family as
they would influence the patient's choice; (4) the possibility of adverse
side effects; (5) prognosis without treatment, again as it might influence the patient's choice; and (6) the prognosis with treatment. Thus,
for example, Richard Roe's previous refusal of treatment during his
psychotic decompensation became evidence of his expressed preference.
If this is to be the approach to determining preference, I think it is a
great mistake. The Roe family, for example, is condemned to keep their
psychotic son at home and watch him get sicker and sicker without any
assistance. How long will it be before they abandon him? How long will
it be before the state is hiring bureaucrats to serve as guardians for such
patients? How long will it be before the newspapers are reporting
neglect and abuse by these public guardians? The *Roe* and *Rogers* courts
are locked into a legal conception in which each man is an island. They
see their task as to protect the autonomy of that person. But in the end,
this legal approach may succeed in making its conception the reality.
The person will have become an island.

The Supreme Court in *Parham* rejected the *Bartley v. Kremens*
approach to minors. But by making no distinction between families and
welfare agencies, and by ignoring the problem of dumping and the
quality of the institutions, it in effect ignored what I believe to be other
crucial policy issues.[61]

PSYCHIATRISTS AS POLICEMEN AND DRUG ABUSE

During the past two decades critics of psychiatry have repeatedly
attacked the profession because it played at the same time conflicting
and misleading roles. As therapists, we encourage our patients to speak
with candor and hold nothing back because only in this way can the patient be helped. But, it is said, we also serve a police function and we
have other institutional masters. The legal and ethical consequences of
this double agent behavior were nicely expressed by a cartoonist who
pictures a trusting patient lying on a couch pouring his heart out while
behind him the psychoanalyst is sneaking out of the room and a

policeman is sneaking in. I have argued in all of these essays that this kind of double agentry needs to be explicitly recognized and that with rare exceptions the psychiatrist should come down on the side of being a therapist and eschew police functions.

But law-makers have increasingly taken quite the opposite position. Those who make legal policy have opted for resolving the conflict of roles in favor of making psychiatrists play the role of policemen. This is a red thread that runs through many recent legal developments that touch on the practice of psychiatry. That of course is what the criminalization of civil commitment does: it asks psychiatrists to decide who should be in a hospital and who should be let out, not on therapeutic grounds but on the policeman's criterion of danger to society. As I shall demonstrate, that is even the policy concealed behind the right to refuse treatment. The articulation of this police policy is by no means confined to constitutional litigation. The *Tarasoff*[62] decision—which expanded tort liability by imposing on psychiatrists a duty to protect society— rests, at bottom, on a policy judgment that society is better served by ob- ligating psychotherapists to act as policemen who are to make use of information gained from patients in the expectation of confidentiality. A similar policy judgment underlies statutory provisions requiring the reporting of drug prescriptions; these laws sacrifice the privacy of the doctor-patient relationship to the state's policy interest in monitoring drug abuse. All of these and other legal developments require the psychiatrists to assume police functions. If psychiatrists were in fact effective policemen there might be some rationality in this scheme, but they are not. They have neither science nor clinical widsom to guide their police decisions. Furthermore, each new conflict between the therapeutic and the police role eats away at the fundamental ethical position of the profession. One of the least obvious but most important examples of this is the right to refuse treatment.

The right to refuse treatment has been conceptualized by the federal district courts as follows: to move from a condition of confine- ment to confinement plus forced treatment with antipsychotic medica- tion is to move across a constitutionally protected line. One theory of the constitutional claim is that the protected line marks the zone of privacy. A second theory is that the antipsychotic drugs violate one's First Amendment rights by altering the brain, the mind, and thus mentation, speech, and thought.[63] Both of these theories, it seems to me, require at least that all forced drug treatment, and not just treatment with antipsychotic drugs, be deemed a constitutional violation. It is a strange conception of privacy that distinguishes between the contents of different syringes. If an injection of Thorazine is a violation of privacy, then it would seem that so is an injection of Valium. Furthermore, the notion that the antipsychotic drugs are mind-altering in a way that other drugs in the psychiatric armamentarium are not is simply incorrect. None of these drugs will change Democrats into Republicans. On the other hand, all of them either directly or indirectly alter the chemistry of the brain. Chief Justice Hennessey of the Massachusetts Supreme Judicial Court, who wrote the *Richard Roe III* opinion, described the side effects of antipsychotic drugs as "frequently devastating and often irreversible." He was particularly and explicitly concerned about the principal side effect—tardive dyskinesia. He went so far as to suggest in a footnote that if an antipsychotic without side effects were discovered it might lead him to revise his judicial opinion.[64] Side effects also seem to have played a crucial role in other constitutional right-to-refuse treatment decisions, including the Massachusetts Supreme Judicial Court's final resolution of *Rogers v. Commissioner*.[65] But if side effects are the crucial consideration, then what these judges are really saying has less to do with privacy or the First Amendment and more to do with their assessments of the risks and benefits of antipsychotic medication. Indeed the singling out of antipsychotic medication is what gives the right to refuse treatment decisions the quality Justice Stewart described—that is, they are serious problems of policy disguised as questions of constitutional law.

If we go back to the original formulation which seems so powerful and convincing (the line between confinement and confinement plus treatment) and look more carefully, we discover that, although the rhetoric dealt with individual autonomy, it is also another way of announcing the fundamental principle of criminalization—namely, that the only justification for confinement of the mentally ill is the protection of society. Once the patient is confined, society's need is satisfied and the state has no compelling reason to treat the patient. The right to refuse treatment is, in a sense, a compromise between society's police interest in security and the patient's right to be mad. This reasoning of course simply rejects *parens patriae* and assigns to the mental hospital the role of jail and to its staff the role of policemen. This is what I mean by the red thread that runs through much recent mental health litigation. Where the psychiatrist has played the two often-conflicting roles of therapist and policeman, the courts have for a variety of reasons as in the right to refuse treatment resolved the conflict by forcing the psychiatrist into the role of policeman.

This police policy was a critical question in *Rogers v. Okin* and in other cases. (As the Massachusetts commissioners of Mental Health changed, so has the name of the case: from *Rogers v. Macht* to *Rogers v. Okin* to *Rogers v. Mills* to the final generic *Rogers v. Commissioner of Mental Health*.) The court was asked to consider what constitutes an emergency in which the state can impose antipsychotic drugs on a patient who otherwise has a right to refuse treatment. Chief Justice Hennessey of the Massachusetts court had looked to the dictionary for a definition of medical emergency. He had decided that Richard Roe's deterioration into chronic schizophrenia was not an emergency. Judge Tauro of the federal court decided that such an emergency existed for committed patients only when there was "a substantial likelihood of physical harm to that patient, other patients, or to staff."[66]

Obviously Judge Tauro has adopted a police power standard: when a crime of violence against persons is about to be committed, an emergency exists. The police, of course, would have a duty to intervene even to prevent lesser crimes, like sexual molestation and destruction of property, the "crimes" repeatedly committed by named plaintiffs in *Rogers v. Okin*.[67] But Judge Tauro does not believe that every emergency which justifies police intervention justifies emergency treatment. The principle, of course, is that a high threshold is necessary to protect the patient's individual autonomy or, put differently, the patient's right to be mad in a manner short of violence. But the question must arise, what about the other patients who are the victims of these nonviolent crimes? Must they simply endure a lawless community like those that exist in our jails and prisons? Psychiatrists have found that when they attempt to have hospitalized patients prosecuted for any crime short of murder, the district attorney's office is unwilling to proceed. The patients are too sick to be prosecuted, but they are not sick enough to be treated.

I am confident that if Judge Tauro saw a man breaking up the furniture in his courtroom or spray painting graffiti on the walls he would call a policeman to stop what was happening. He might even order him arrested or sent to a mental hospital. Does the fact that the offender has already been confined in a mental hospital mean he now has a right to subject the patients and the staff to that same offensive behavior? I have worked in wards that were run by patient government, where patients made the rules, and it is clear to me that mental patients are no more immune to and no less offended by such antisocial actions than are nonpatients. They do not want the only television set broken, the dinner table turned over, or patients running about naked. Indeed, such offensive behavior is even more appalling because the patient cannot escape it by going home. Ironically it is because the psychiatrist

is concerned about these issues that the Supreme Judicial Court of
Massachusetts which finally decided the *Rogers* case declared he has an
unacceptable conflict of interests.[68]

The judge may be correct in thinking that since the public has been
protected by involuntary confinement, society as a whole has no further
interest in such "crazy behavior." But the other patients in the ward do
have a continuing interest. A balance must be struck not only between
society's interests and those of an individual patient, but also between
that patient and the other patients who are confined with him. These
are, of course, complicated matters, but they are real problems to which
the courts have been quite insensitive, partly because as in *Rogers v.
Mills* the lawyers are allowed the legal fiction of claiming that they
represent the entire class of patients. Thus important conflicts among
the interests of different patients get glossed over.[69]

But my major objection to Judge Tauro's standard for emergency
involuntary antipsychotic drug treatment is not just the level of his
police power threshold which transforms mental hospitals back into
madhouses. Rather it seems to me that his entire conception is flawed.
Substantial likelihood of physical harm is not an appropriate medical
criterion for emergency antipsychotic medication. Much of the violence
on psychiatric wards is not caused by psychotic patients. Donna Hunt,
for example, one of the named plaintiffs in *Rogers v. Okin*, had a
behavior disorder and was mentally retarded as a consequence of
childhood encephalitis.[70] Antipsychotic drugs for such patients are not
appropriate medical treatment. Violence, even on psychiatric wards, is
often created by patients who, although they have a diagnosable mental
illness, are competent to make treatment decisions. When a psychiatrist
administers treatment to a patient in the face of a competent refusal, he
is not acting as an ethical physician. He is nothing but an agent of police
control. If the "treatment" is a single injection of a short-acting
antipsychotic drug, it hardly deserves to be called treatment no matter
what the patient's diagnosis may be. The question for a doctor is
whether the "crazy behavior" is a manifestation of a mental illness that
responds to antipsychotic medication.

Judge Tauro has articulated not a medical standard for emergency
treatment, but a police standard for the use of antipsychotic drugs as
chemical restraint. Psychiatrists who follow that standard act as policemen.

There is still more wrong with this approach to the right to refuse
antipsychotic drugs, but I shall emphasize here only one concern which

it seems has been ignored. The most abused drugs in the world today are the minor tranquilizers (Valium, Librium, etc).[71] They are enormously overprescribed; unlike the antipsychotic drugs, they are reinforcing and, in large quantities, addictive. As I have noted before, the overprescription of these drugs has been one of the great medical scandals of our society. Yet the *Roe* and the *Rogers v. Mills* decisions, by limiting the use of antipsychotic drugs even in appropriate cases, create an incentive for psychiatrists to administer minor tranquilizers to their psychotic patients.

One may justly object that no court is *requiring* doctors to prescribe inappropriate drugs, but in reality psychiatrists do prescribe them, and these judicial decisions constitute a regulatory incentive to still more of this inappropriate treatment. Moreover, these decisions make these less effective, addictive drugs appropriate by limiting access to other drugs which in many cases are medically preferable. Nor is this merely a hypothetical matter. Before antipsychotics became available, psychiatrists prescribed minor tranquilizers for profoundly anxious psychotic patients in the absence of anything better. Now, with access to antipsychotics limited, psychiatrists will once again have to rely on less effective drugs. The judges, in their version of constitutional or police wisdom, have in this and other respects simply turned the clock back twenty-five years. The judges have done all this in an effort to protect the patient's autonomy. To accomplish that end, they have restricted the psychiatrist's therapeutic discretion. Their approach to limiting discretion may result in very sick patients being deprived of effective treatment, but almost as bad in my view, it requires psychiatrists to think like policemen.

CONCLUSION

No doubt, as you were warned at the outset, there has been overstatement in all this. I have not even mentioned what I think has been good and just about psychiatric and legal reform. I have tried to do that elsewhere in these essays. For the empiricists and those who struggle with multiple regression analysis, this will have been quite unsatisfactory. I can only hope that I have challenged them to disprove this bill of particulars. As for legal activists who believe theirs is a sacred cause, I have offended their faith with my agnosticism. I can only hope to have shaken their sense of certainty. In the views of psychiatrists who believe that some things are best left unsaid, I will have violated professional etiquette. I can only remind them that professional etiquette is not professional responsibility.

In the end I stand by my bill of particulars, because on reflection I see that these claims have a common theme. The cunning of modern bureaucracy is that it creates a hierarchy in which no one feels personally responsible for anything important that goes wrong. Every-where I look I see the public mental health system being shaped by this cunning, and legal reform seems to me to have hastened that process. By setting barriers in the path of treatment responsibilities, and by imposing on psychiatrists responsibilities they could not fulfill, legal reform has turned a ratchet that will not easily be turned back. As we pass through the 1980s the great ideological dragon of psychiatry has been coaxed out of its cave. The major legal battles have been fought, and when the dust settled the dragon was gone and all that remained was a collection of hapless civil servants. Yet madness has not gone out of the world as was hoped, in fact madness is more visible than ever before in this century. One can see chronic mental patients in the streets of every major city in the United States. These painful realities have taken much of the glamour out of law and psychiatry, the great civil libertarian crusade is over. Perhaps with fewer illusions about law and about psychiatry, those of us who still care can attempt the difficult task of a new beginning.

REFERENCES

1. *Parham v. J. R.*, 442 U.S. 584, 624–625 (1979).

2. Stone, Response to the Presidential Address, *American Journal of Psychiatry*, Vol. 136, pp. 1020–1022 (August 1979).

3. 412 F.Supp. 112 (1976).

4. 95 S.Ct. 2486 (1975).

5. 99 S.Ct. 1804 (1979).

6. *Schweiker v. Wilson*, 101 S.Ct. 1074 (1981).

7. *See, e.g., Suzuki v. Quisenberry*, 411 F.Supp. 1113 (D.C.Hawaii 1976), and *Lessard v. Schmidt*, 349 F.Supp. 1078 (E.D.Wis. 1972).

8. *See* Surveys of state law and theories of civil commitment, Developments in the Law, Civil Commitment of the Mentally Ill, *Harvard Law Review*, Vol. 87, pp. 1190–1406 (1974) and Legal Issues in State Mental Health Care: Proposals for Change, Civil Commitment, *Mental Disability Law Reporter*, Vol. 2, pp. 75–126 (July–August 1977).

9. *See, e.g.*, the discussion of California's Lanterman-Petris-Short Act (Cal. Welf. & Inst'ns Code §§5000-401) in A. Stone, *Mental Health and Law: A System in Transition* (National Institute of Mental Health, 1975), pp. 60–65.

10. *See, e.g.*, Committed Mental Patients Stroll Out to Freedom, *New York Times*, January 9, 1981, p. B1.

11. *See* Note, Plea Bargaining and the Transformation of the Criminal Process, *Harvard Law Review*, Vol. 90, p. 564 (1977). In 1975, 31,170 of the 48,244 cases filed in federal district courts were disposed of by guilty pleas. *Ibid.*

12. *See, e.g.*, Brooklyn Office Decides the Treatment of Cases That Involve a Felony Charge, *New York Times*, January 4, 1981, p. 78.

13. *See*, 99% of Felony Arrests in the City Fail to Bring Terms in State Prison, *New York Times*, January 4, 1981, p. 1.

14. See the essay on the trial of John Hinckley (Chapter IV).

15. 406 U.S. 715 (1972).

16. *See, e.g.*, Wisconsin Statutes Annotated 975.06.

17. *See Bolton v. Harris*, 395 F.2d 642 (D.C. Cir. 1968).

18. *See, e.g.*, N.Y. Crim. Pro. Law §330.20.

19. Presented in Pasework, Pantle, and Steadman, Characteristics and Disposition of Persons Found Not Guilty by Reason of Insanity in New York State, 1971–1976, *American Journal of Psychiatry*, Vol. 136, pp. 655–660 (1979).

20. See the summary of Dershowitz's views in Stone, *Mental Health and Law, op. cit.*, pp. 4–8.

21. *Ibid.*, p. 43.

22. *Suzuki v. Quisenberry*, 411 F.Supp. 1113.

23. Quoted in Stone, *op. cit.*, p. 36.

24. *See, e.g.*, N.Y. Crim. Pro. Law §730.60.

25. *Bolton v. Harris*, 395 F. 2d 642.

26. *Suzuki v. Quisenberry*, 411 F.Supp. 1113.

27. *See* state guided-discretion statutes, e.g. Tex. Code Crim. Pro. Art. 37.071 (Vernon Supp. 1980).

28. *See, e.g.*, Ennis and Litwack, Psychiatry and the Presumption of Expertise: Flipping Coins in the Courtroom, *California Law Review*, Vol. 63, pp. 671, 750 (1974).

29. Monahan, Prediction Research and the Emergency Commitment of Dangerous Mentally Ill Persons: A Reconsideration, *American Journal of Psychiatry*, Vol. 135, pp. 198–201 (1978).

30. S. Halleck, *Psychiatry and the Dilemmas of Crime: A Study of Causes, Punishment and Treatment* (University of California Press, 1971).

31. *See, e.g., Jurek v. Texas*, 428 U.S.262, 274–276.

32. *See* N. Ridenour, *Mental Health in the United States: A Fifty-Year History* (1961); Beiser, Psychiatric Epidemiology, in A. M. Nicholi, *Harvard Guide to Modern Psychiatry* (Harvard University Press, 1978), pp. 609–626; L. Bellak and H. Barton, *Progress in Community Mental Health* (Basic Books, 1975).

33. L. Bellak, *Schizophrenia: A Review of the Syndrome* (Basic Books, 1958), p. 75.

34. Stone, *op. cit.*, p. 41.

35. J. J. Paris, The New York Court of Appeals Rules on the Rights of Incompetent Dying Patients, *New England Journal of Medicine*, Vol. 304, pp. 1424–1425 (1981).

36. *See* Judge Tauro's explanation of the Massachusetts seclusion statute (Mass. G. L. Ann. Ch. 123, §21) in *Rogers v. Okin*, 478 F.Supp. 1342, 1371–1372 (1979).

37. *See* Appelbaum and Gutheil, "Rotting With Their Rights on": Constitutional Theory and Clinical Reality in Drug Refusal by Psychiatric Patients, *Bulletin of the American Academy of Psychiatry and Law*, Vol. 7, p. 308–317 (1979); and Stone, Recent Mental Health Litigation: A Critical Perspective, *American Journal of Psychiatry*, Vol. 134, pp. 273–279 (1977).

38. *See In the Matter of Guardianship of Richard Roe, III* Mass. Adv. Sh. (1981) 981.

39. Mass. General Laws Annotated, Ch. 766.

40. *In the Matter of Guardianship of Roe*, Mass. Adv. Sh. (1981) 981, 986.

41. *Rogers v. Okin*, 478 F. Supp 1342.

42. Patterson, Perspective, *The Journal of the Denver General Hospital* (Fall 1980).

43. *See* R. Rock, M. Jakobson, and R. Janopaul, *Hospitalization and Discharge of the Mentally Ill* (1968). *See also* Hardisty, Mental Illness: A Legal Fiction, *Washington Law Review*, Vol. 48, pp.735–762 (1973).

44. *See generally* J. Talbott, *The Death of the Asylum: A Critical Study of State Hospital Management, Services, and Care* (Grune and Stratton, 1978).

45. *See* U. E. Reinhardt, *Physican Productivity and the Demand for Health Manpower* (1975); and Group for the Advancement of Psychiatry, *The Effect of Method of Payment on Mental Health and Practice* (1975).

46. Sharfstein and Clark, Why Psychiatry Is a Low-Paid Medical Specialty, *American Journal of Psychiatry*, Vol. 137, pp. 831–833 (1980).

47. Stone, The Myth of Advocacy, *Hospital and Community Psychiatry* Vol. 30, pp. 819–823 (1979).

48. Torrey and Taylor, Cheap Labor from Poor Nations, *American Journal of Psychiatry*, Vol. 130, pp. 428–433 (1973).

49. 644 F. 2d 147 (1980).

50. *Ibid.*, p. 185 (Aldisert, Circuit Judge, dissenting).

51. A. B. Hollingshead and F. C. Redlich, *Social Class and Mental Illness: A Community Study* (Wiley, 1958).

52. *See* Meissner and Nicholi, Jr., The Psychotherapies: Individual, Family, and Group, in *Harvard Guide to Modern Psychiatry, supra*, pp. 357–386.

53. 402 F.Supp. 1039 (E.D.Pa. 1975); judgment vacated *sub. nom. Kremens v. Bartley*, 431 U.S. 119 (1977).

54. 402 F.Supp. 1039, 1053.

55. *Ibid.*, pp. 1047–1048.

56. Mass. Adv. Sh. (1981) 981, 1087.

57. *See, e.g., In re Boyd*, 403 A.2d 744 (DC 1979) at 749.

58. *Ibid.*

59. *See, e.g.*, Utah Code Ann. 64-7-36 (10) (Supp. 79) and *A. E. and R. R. v. Mitchell*, No. 78-466 (D. Utah 1980); discussed in Stone, The Right to Refuse Treatment: Why Psychiatrists Should and Can Make It Work, *Archives of General Psychiatry*, Vol. 38, p. 362 (1981).

60. *See In the Matter of Guardianship of Roe*, Mass. Adv. Sh. (1981) at 1012–13. *Rogers v. Commissioner of Mental Health*, 390 Mass. 489 (1983).

61. Justices Brennan, Marshall, and Stevens showed more awareness of these issues. See *Parham v. J. R.*, 422 U.S. 584, 625–639 (Brennan, J. concurring in part and dissenting in part).

62. *Tarasoff v. Regents of the University of California*, 529 P.2d 553 (1974).

63. *See* Stone, The Right to Refuse Treatment, *op. cit.*, p. 59.

64. *In the Matter of Guardianship of Richard Roe, III*, Mass. Adv. Sh. (1981) 981, l006n.

65. *Rogers v. Commissioner of Mental Health*, 390 Mass. 489.

66. *Rogers v. Okin*, 478 F.Supp. 1342 (D. Mass. 1979), 1159–1160.

67. *Rogers v. Okin*, 478 F.Supp. 1342, 1365.

68. *Rogers v. Commissioner of Mental Health*, 390 Mass. 489 at 503. *See Rogers v. Okin, Ibid.*, at 1379–1380.

69. In principle, Federal Rule of Civil Procedure 23(b)(3) should ensure that federal courts do not certify classes of plaintiffs the members of which have conflicting interests. The first time *Kremens v. Bartley* reached the Supreme Court, the Court declined to decide the case as it was then constituted as a class action. The Court noted "very possible differences in the interests of different members of the class," and remanded the case to the district court after vacating its judgment. 431 U.S. 119, 135–137 (1977).

70. *Rogers v. Okin*, 478 F.Supp. at 1354.

71. J. Marks, *The Benzodiazepines: Use, Overuse, Misuse, Abuse* (University Park Press, 1978).

VII

The *Tarasoff* Case and Some of Its Progeny: Suing Psychotherapists to Safeguard Society

ON OCTOBER 27, 1969, Prosenjit Poddar, a citizen of India studying naval architecture at the University of California at Berkeley, shot and stabbed to death Tatiana Tarasoff, a young woman with whom he had had a casual acquaintance. He had psychotically elaborated their relationship in his own mind so that it had become of enormous significance. He made her the center of his emotional life; she became the primary ambivalent figure. Loved and hated, all good and all evil, he killed her because she had rejected his love.

Poddar, like John Hinckley, seems to have been a candidate for the diagnosis of erotomania or Clerambault's syndrome. Poddar was convicted of voluntary manslaughter and confined to the Vacaville facility.[1] He has since been released from prison, has returned to India, and by his own account is now happily married.[2] The remedies of the criminal justice system have been exhausted, but the tragedy of Miss Tarasoff's death has set off a legal imbroglio in the civil courts that has and will proliferate during the decade of the 1980s and that involves anyone who might be described as a psychotherapist.

THE *TARASOFF* CASE

The facts of *Tarasoff v. Regents of the University of California*,[3] seem to be as follows. Poddar sought psychiatric assistance as an outpatient at the student health facility at Berkeley and was evaluated by a psychiatrist, who referred Poddar to a psychologist for psychotherapy. The psychologist subsequently decided that Poddar was dangerous. This judgment was not based on any arcane clinical judgment. Poddar had revealed his pathological attachment to Tatiana Tarasoff, and the psychologist had been told by a friend of Poddar's that he intended to purchase a gun. The psychologist therefore, quite responsibly, first consulted with psychiatric colleagues and then notified the campus police at Berkeley both orally and in writing that Poddar was mentally ill and dangerous and should be taken by the campus police to a facility authorized under California's civil commitment statute to commit him. These steps are envisioned under the provisions of California's civil commitment statute.[4] California, unlike most other states,[5] now limits the legal authority of private psychiatrists to authorize emergency involuntary confinement.

The police interviewed Poddar at length and independently concluded that he was rational and not dangerous. They decided not to take him to a committing facility after he promised to stay away from Miss Tarasoff, who was then in Brazil. They reported their actions to the clinic. Up to this point in the story, it is difficult to find anything resembling negligence on the part of the psychotherapists. If anyone behaved improperly, it was the police who made an independent judgment about the likelihood of Poddar's violence and his sanity and rejected the judgment of the clinic.

The psychiatrist in charge of the clinic, who had been absent during these events, returned and apparently decided that his staff had overreacted. In the name of confidentiality, he requested that the police return the correspondence about Poddar and ordered that it and other records of the therapy be destroyed. He also allegedly directed that no further action be taken to detain or commit Poddar.

If this account is correct, then it presents the first instance of professional conduct which might be considered negligent. The psychiatrist's actions certainly seem odd, if not negligent. But much of this account is based on allegations, and much is left to conjecture. It is unclear whether the director of the clinic simply put more faith in the judgment of the police than in that of his own staff, or why he felt it necessary to destroy the records.[6] At any rate, Poddar, understandably, never returned for psychotherapy. And it is unclear whether the clinic made any further efforts to contact him.

While Tatiana Tarasoff was out of the country during the summer, Poddar broke his promise to the police and established a relationship with her brother. The brother, allegedly not having been warned, was unaware of the danger Poddar posed. On Miss Tarasoff's return to the country some two months after Poddar's encounters with the psycho-therapist and the campus police, he went to her home and killed her.

Miss Tarasoff's parents attempted to sue the Regents of the University of California, the therapist involved, and the police. The trial court dismissed the complaint, holding that, despite the tragic events, there was no legal basis in the law of California for a claim against them.[7] After the dismissal was affirmed by the court of appeal, the parents' lawyers appealed to the Supreme Court of California, arguing that the judges should hold that the defendants had had a duty to warn Miss Tarasoff or her family of the danger and that they had also had a duty to bring about Poddar's confinement under the provisions of California's Lanterman-Petris-Short civil commitment statute.[8] This distinction between the duty to warn and the duty to commit was to be crucial not only for the *Tarasoff* decision but also for all of the subsequent cases for which *Tarasoff* was a precedent.

If the courts had held in 1973 that psychiatrists have a duty to commit in order to avoid personal liability, that decision would have run counter to the thrust of legal reform which was making involuntary confinement much more difficult.

In the first of its two decisions in *Tarasoff*, the California Supreme Court reversed the dismissal,[9] finding that the *special relationship* of the therapists to the patient had given them a duty to warn Miss Tarasoff. In addition, the court held that the police might be liable for a failure to warn on the theory that their abortive attempt to commit Poddar involuntarily had deterred him from seeking further therapy and aggra-vated the danger to Miss Tarasoff. *Tarasoff I* stood for the proposition that psychotherapists and the police in such a situation have a duty to warn—not a duty to commit.

The defendants, joined by several *amici curiae*, petitioned for rehearing, which the court, in an unusual step, granted.[10] In its second decision, without attempting to explain—and without even mention-ing—its original opinion, the court abandoned its position on the liability of police. The opinion stated only that the police did not have a *special relationship* with either Poddar or the victim that was sufficient to give rise to a duty to warn. The result is ironic given the facts of the

Tarasoff case and the crucial role the police had played. Of course, as the State of California had argued in an *amicus* brief, the consequences of creating negligence liability for police every time they are involved with a potentially dangerous person would have enormous implications, financial and otherwise. But given the court's derivation of the "special relationship," it is absurd that therapists have one and the police do not.

The second *Tarasoff* opinion formulated the duty of the therapists more broadly, holding that the special relationship between a therapist and patient imposes on the therapist a duty to use reasonable care to protect third parties against danger posed by the patient. Whether this duty takes the form of a duty to warn, a duty to call the police, or some other form, will depend—in a way the court did not attempt to clarify—on the circumstances.

In the circumstances of *Tarasoff*, the court held, the plaintiffs might allege that the duty to protect took the form of a duty to warn. These duties, in *Tarasoff II* terms, are all predicated on the special relationship of therapist to patient. The Tarasoff family settled their claim out of court and thus we do not know whether a judge or jury would have found negligence in this landmark case. But new law had been set down and new duties imposed on therapists. Other jurisdictions would thereafter look to the California precedent. California is well known for its legal innovations.

THE THEORY BEHIND *TARASOFF*

Both *Tarasoff* decisions were strongly influenced by an article by John Fleming and Bruce Maximov,[11] published while the case was on appeal to the California Supreme Court. The article is typical of much law review literature of the past two decades in its critical assault on psychiatric decisionmaking. The neutral tone of the article is deceptive, for its legal conclusions rely heavily on the evaluation of the psychiatric profession made by the small group of radical critics of psychiatry led by Doctor Thomas Szasz.

Doctor Szasz opposes all involuntary psychiatric intervention and has characterized such intervention as the "manufacture of madness."[12] His views have been embraced by some legal reformers, and he is regularly cited by them as the authority on psychiatry in law review articles and civil libertarian briefs. His views have thus found their way into judicial opinions.

This perspective on psychiatry frames Fleming and Maximov's

consideration of the dilemma faced by a therapist who "believes" that a patient under his or her treatment poses a serious threat to a third party. The origin of Fleming and Maximov's conception of the therapist's new affirmative duty is indicated by the title of their article, "The Patient or His Victim: The Therapist's Dilemma."

The authors argue that, on the one hand, the therapist has an obligation to maintain the patient's confidences given in therapy, and that the patient, *even if* believed to be dangerous, has an interest in privacy, liberty, and due process. These factors mitigate against the therapist's acting to protect third parties by committing the patient, even when the therapist believes the patient is seriously mentally ill and dangerous—that is *even when committable* under most state laws. But concern for public safety makes some action imperative. The problem the authors faced, given their libertarian ideology, was in defining what legal obligation other than civil commitment could be placed on the psychotherapist.

Tort law traditionally had held that an ordinary citizen has no duty to warn a third party. Thus, if I am standing on a corner and I see a blind man about to step in front of an oncoming bus, I have no duty to warn him. But Fleming and Maximov argued that the therapeutic relationship was sufficiently "special" under the principles of tort law to overcome this rule of nonfeasance and so to allow policy considerations to determine the duty of the therapist.

The "therapist's dilemma" is to be resolved by balancing the interests of society against the interests of the patient. But the therapist cannot be trusted to perform that balancing, for it cannot be assumed that he or she will sufficiently safeguard the interests of the patient he or she believes to be dangerous. Indeed, Fleming and Maximov see the gravest risks to the patient as coming from coercive legal decisions of the therapist, such as the decision to commit Poddar.

In following the normal course of involuntarily committing a patient, "the psychiatrist in many instances serves not only as arresting officer, but as prosecutor, judge, and jailer as well."[13] Relying on the radical critics of psychiatry, the authors assume that commitment is the worst thing that the psychiatrist can do to his patient. It deprives him of liberty, stigmatizes him, destroys his will to resist, and breaches confidentiality.

Thus the dilemma faced by the conscientious therapist, according to Fleming and Maximov, is how to protect the public without abusing psychiatry's awesome preemption of legal authority through involuntary commitment. Their resolution is to place on the therapist the duty to protect society in the manner least harmful to the interests of the patient.[14] That duty, they believe, will vary from case to case and will often take the form of a duty to warn potential victims.

The breach of confidentiality required by a duty to warn such parties, the authors imply, is far preferable to the abusive and customary alternative of confining the patient. Fleming and Maximov make no attempt to consider the protective value to victims of a telephone warning from a psychotherapist. Nor do they respond to the argument that such warnings do not protect society as much as would confine ment of the patient. The duty they impose is designed as much to protect patients from the power of psychiatrists as to protect the public from dangerous patients.

It must be emphasized that these authors were asserting that the preferable course of action is to allow a patient like Poddar, who has been diagnosed as mentally ill and dangerous, to go free so long as his vic tim or victims have been warned. So much were they concerned about the discretionary authority of psychiatry, and so little were they concerned about public safety. Thus, recalling the original *Tarasoff* complaint that there was either a duty to warn or a duty to confine, Fleming and Maximov came down strongly on the duty to warn. Clearly they did not want to create new legal incentives (the threat of civil liability) for civil commitment. They had found a new legal application of the principle of the least restrictive alternative for the "alleged patient."

While the legal and social policy arguments made by Fleming and Maximov have serious shortcomings, the authors at least make an explicit and coherent attempt to balance the interests of the supposedly dangerous patient and of society. Despite the influence of the article on the two *Tarasoff* decisions, however, there is little evidence in either decision of any recognition that the duty to warn the victim is based on a policy of protecting the rights of supposedly dangerous patients.

The decisions in *Tarasoff I* and *Tarasoff II* focused almost entirely on the issue of public safety. The governing factor seemed to be Justice Tobriner's admonition that "[i]n this risk-infested society we can hardly tolerate the further exposure to danger that would result from a concealed knowledge of the therapist that his patient was lethal. . . . The containment of such risks lies in the public interest."[15] On this basis, and after a brief consideration of tort law precedent that relied heavily on Fleming and Maximov, the court held that the existence of a therapist-patient relationship is sufficient to overcome the general presumption against imposing a duty to warn another of a third person's potentially dangerous conduct.

The psychotherapist is special. Unlike the ordinary citizen, he has a duty to warn the blind man that he is about to step in front of a bus. But as we shall see, everything is infinitely more complicated than this simple analogy suggests. Having eliminated the force of the general presumption, the court turned to a consideration of policy and after only a perfunctory balancing of the interests of the patient in privacy and the public in effective treatment concluded that the psychiatrist has a duty to protect third parties that may take the form of warning the potential victim.[16] In so ruling, the court rejected the argument presented by the American Psychiatric Association as *amicus*, that a psychiatrist cannot predict dangerousness with sufficient reliability to make reasonable a duty to protect others from dangerous conduct.

This unreliability on the side of overprediction of dangerousness, which results in a large number of "false positives," stems from the combination of the inevitable element of error involved in psychological predictions with the low "base rate" (that is, rarity) of violent behavior among the mentally ill. The problem has been illustrated as follows:

> Assume that one person out of a thousand will kill. Assume also an exceptionally accurate test is created which differentiates with ninety-five percent effectiveness those who will kill from those who will not. If 100,000 people were tested, out of the 100 who would kill, ninety-five would be isolated. Unfortunately, out of the 99,900 who would not kill, 4,995 people would also be isolated as potential killers.[17]

The point psychiatrists make is that they do not know when a patient will become a bus bearing down on a hapless victim. They emphasize the problems of false positives and overprediction which complicate the court's simple assumption of some "concealed knowledge" that "a patient is lethal."

The court's response to the problems of prediction was, from a legal perspective, simple: the therapist will be expected to display only "that reasonable degree of skill, knowledge, and care ordinarily possessed and exercised by members of [that professional specialty]."[18] The court did not stop to inquire what sense this test makes when no member of the profession can reliably predict dangerousness.[19] Nor did it consider that whenever a law suit is brought, it will be because the therapist's prediction was wrong, and the plaintiff's experts will be looking back with the wisdom of hindsight. If in foresight psychiatrists are unable to predict dangerousness, in hindsight everything seems inevitable—the dangerous patient was lethal.

The court also did not consider whether the kind of breach of confidentiality it endorsed, given the problem of overprediction, would accord with the legitimate expectations of the patient. Nor did it consider potential consequences for the nature of the therapist-patient relationship, and ultimately for the safety of the public. Indeed, Fleming and Maximov's basic concern for the rights of the dangerous patient and their emphasis on the duty to warn as often being the least restrictive alternative for the patient was reduced by the court to little more than a footnote.[20]

TARASOFF I VERSUS TARASOFF II

Where *Tarasoff I* stood for the proposition that psychotherapists and police have a duty to warn third parties who are in danger, *Tarasoff II*— apparently for political reasons—eliminated the police from the picture and at the same time expanded the psychotherapist's duties to third parties. The Tarasoff family's lawyers had asked in *Tarasoff I* that there be liability either for failure to warn an endangered person or for failure to commit the patient who posed the danger. The court, following Fleming and Maximov's result but not their reasoning, came down squarely on the side of the duty to warn.

The American Psychiatric Association, together with its California branches, as noted, attacked this duty to warn both because of the limitations upon accurate predictions of future violence and because of potentially serious inroads upon therapist-patient confidentiality. But the duty to warn was at least a clear and specific obligation from a legal perspective. Ironically, if the duty to warn was originally intended to protect the patient against the psychotherapist, it also protected the psychotherapist by limiting the scope of liability. While psychotherapists objected to the duty to warn in *Tarasoff I*, they got something worse, as subsequent cases have shown.

Tarasoff II made the psychotherapist's duty much less clear. A duty to protect third parties will in some circumstances require a warning, but the court left open what other responsibilities a therapist might have. Although the court did not specify a duty to commit, it could be argued that the duty to protect was perhaps ambiguous enough to include that.

In essence, originally asked to chose between a duty to warn and a duty to confine, the court opted for a third and more ambiguous choice, a duty to protect. Thus they avoided taking a position that would seem to favor civil commitment. But as a result, *Tarasoff II* set a much more ambiguous precedent than did *Tarasoff I*—an ambiguity that would allow ingenious lawyers to claim negligence whenever a patient who has seen a psychotherapist subsequently harms a third party. The central ambiguity of *Tarasoff II* is that it tells the psychotherapist that he or she must protect third parties, but does not specify what steps are legally necessary and sufficient to meet this obligation to protect the public.

Much of the commentary on *Tarasoff*, and even subsequent judicial decisions, have failed to note this distinction. Psychiatrists are still talking about the *Tarasoff* duty to warn, and so are judges. But *Tarasoff II* is the law, and it stands for the duty to protect—a much broader obligation than a narrow duty to warn, and one that creates a much greater risk of liability for psychotherapists.

For example, a duty to warn can logically be applied only to a foreseeable victim. The psychotherapist cannot be liable for not warn-ing unforeseeable victims, as courts have noted. But if the psychothera-pist's duty is to protect third parties, warning in cases when the victim is foreseeable and taking some other unspecified action when the victim is not foreseeable, the scope of liability expands in ways not yet determined, as the following cases will make clear. Consider the patient who goes berserk and starts shooting people in a bar. If the therapist's duty is to protect society, every victim can sue. If his duty is to warn foreseeable victims, none of these third party victims can sue.

Adding to the complexity of *Tarasoff II*'s ambiguous duties is the additional problem of what standards will govern the courts' evaluation of the therapist's performance of those duties.

Judge Mosk, both in his separate opinion in *Tarasoff II* and later, in *Hedlund v. The Superior Court of Orange County*,[21] was concerned about the way the majority had dealt with the psychotherapist's ability to predict dangerousness. Mosk had authored an earlier California Supreme Court opinion that rejected the value of psychiatric testimony as to future dangerousness. He and the court had decided that psychi-atric predictions about future dangerousness were too unreliable as evidence to meet the standard of proof beyond a reasonable doubt that leads to confinement of sexually dangerous persons.[22]

Mosk's views on the subject are now generally accepted by legal reformers. The newly promulgated standards of the American Bar

Association would disallow psychiatric testimony predicting future violent behavior. The ABA's discussion of this issue is consistent with the emerging psychiatric consensus.

Psychiatrists evaluating the mental status of a patient have some expertise in determining whether at that time the patient manifests violent-propensities. However, they cannot predict beyond that present mental status to future violent behavior with any degree of reliability that might be considered a professional skill. This distinction between immediate evaluation allowing expert judgment about imminent vio-lence and prediction of violence beyond that point has been accepted by many clinicians. However, there is still no solid evidence about the reliability of even the immediate evaluations.[23] These considerations do not seem as yet to have influenced judicial opinion on the *Tarasoff* question.

It seemed inconsistent to Mosk for the California Supreme Court to reject the value of such professional efforts when given in court but to accept this expertise as a standard of care in the therapist's office for imposing liability on psychotherapists. If the ABA's standards are accepted, the lawmakers will in effect have so discredited the ability of psychotherapists to predict future violence that such testimony will not be admissible even in a court that is deciding about the confinement of a violent mentally ill offender who has already committed an act of violence.

Yet *Tarasoff* holds the therapist liable for malpractice on the basis of those very same predictions, even without a prior act of violence, as was the case with Poddar. That result is absurd. The only tenable justification for this absurdity is the understandable desire to compen-sate victims by reaching into the therapists' malpractice policy in order to find a deep pocket.

Mosk saw the issue in *Tarasoff* as whether a psychotherapist should be expected to have some special professional capacity to predict dangerousness. If so, when the prediction is wrong, the psychotherapist should be judged by the traditional "standard of care" as delineated in medical malpractice cases. This standard of care is held to demand "that reasonable degree of knowledge and skill which is ordinarily possessed and exercised by other members of the profession in similar circum-stances."[24]

This standard allows the plaintiff to introduce expert testimony second-guessing a psychotherapist's initial prediction from the wisdom of hindsight. Mosk argued that if the court was consistent, it should concede that therapists have no special expertise and therefore that the malpractice standard, which is predicated on professional expertise, should not be applicable.

Mosk argued that there should be liability only when the therapist has "actual" knowledge of intended violence and can therefore be judged by an ordinary negligence standard. For Mosk, failure to warn a third party once a therapist has actual knowledge of an imminent threat does not involve "medical care or treatment of a patient . . . but [is] a species of civilian duty that has arisen to a third party." Thus, "the acts or omissions of the doctors are not malpractice, but simple negli-gence."[25]

Thus the psychotherapist does have a "species of civilian" duty unlike the ordinary citizen's. But the performance of this duty is not to be judged as if it is based on the arcane knowledge of therapists who are expert at predicting dangerousness and at protecting the public. Only when the therapist actually knows the bus is bearing down on the blind person does he have a duty, and that duty is not that of an expert but that of an ordinary person.

Mosk's discussion of the issue did not take into account the earlier mentioned distinction between evaluation of violence in current mental status and prediction of future behavior. The majority simply assumed professional expertise, and Mosk assumed no professional expertise, in the detection and prediction of future violence.

The distinction between these two paradigms—standard of care malpractice and ordinary negligence—is quite important. If therapists are held to a malpractice standard rather than an ordinary negligence standard, not only can their failure to predict violence be second-guessed, but anything that a therapist fails to do when evaluating a patient's dangerousness is potentially negligent as well—particularly when judged in retrospect by the plaintiff's experts, as subsequent cases make clear.

In addition to an actual failure to warn, then, the failure to perform a "sufficient" investigation in order to identify the persons who are "foreseeably" threatened by a patient—and the failure adequately to investigate material that might help one to predict a patient's dangerous-ness—may be deemed actionably negligent. Thus both the application of the malpractice standard and the ambiguous duty to protect expand the potential liability of the therapist. Although one or two jurisdictions have rejected Tarasoff, the trend is toward acceptance of this new legal duty. But there is considerable confusion about the limits of the duty and the different implications of Tarasoff I and Tarasoff II.[26]

AFTER *TARASOFF*

Questions regarding the governing standard for therapists' duties have
been played out in several important decisions since *Tarasoff*. The
concept that negligent malpractice may inhere in the failure of a
therapist to investigate sufficiently to predict dangerousness has received perhaps its greatest notoriety in the context of a suit brought
against John Hinckley's psychiatrists by three men who were seriously
injured in Hinckley's attempt on the President's life.[27]

The United States District Court for the District of Colorado
recently dismissed the complaint that alleged that Hinckley's psychiatrist, Doctor Hopper, had been negligent according to the standards of
his profession (the malpractice standard) in failing to exercise due
diligence in his examination, diagnosis, and treatment of Hinckley.

The plaintiffs relied on psychiatric testimony made during John
Hinckley's trial and charged that Doctor Hopper should have been
aware that Hinckley's behavior—in particular his fascination with the
movie "Taxi Driver" and with books about political assassination—
made the plaintiffs' injuries foreseeable in the event of a "foreseeable"
attack upon the President.

The Colorado court rejected the argument that the existence of a
special therapist-patient relationship creates duties which extend "to
the world at large."[28] "[T]he key issue is to what extent was Doctor
Hopper obligated to protect these particular plaintiffs from this particular harm?"[29] In this case the court held that there was no relationship
between the defendant and the plaintiffs sufficient to create a legal
obligation running from him to them. The decision noted with favor a
rule limiting therapists' duties under *Tarasoff* to situations in which
there have been "specific threats to specific victims."[30] In effect this
court rejected the duty to protect society at large and implicitly opted
for the duty to warn identifiable victims.

But the California courts that decided *Tarasoff* have been receptive to the view that professional standards of care (in traditional
malpractice terms) ought to govern *Tarasoff* duties. The effect of this
view is almost the same as to hold that the therapist has a duty to protect
society at large. Six years after *Tarasoff*, in 1980, *Mavroudis v. The
Superior Court of San Mateo County*[31] refined *Tarasoff* in a manner
that moved in the direction of expanding liability by applying the
malpractice standard. The case centered on pretrial discovery by
petitioners (victims of a violent attack by their son) of their son's
psychiatric records. *Mavroudis* was framed in terms of "whether

various health care providers knew or reasonably should have known the patient presented a serious danger to them."[32]

The *Mavroudis* court concluded that the court below had erred in confining the duties stated in *Tarasoff* to specifically named third parties who are endangered by patients. Instead, *Tarasoff* in their view "stated the duty to use reasonable care to protect the intended victim arises whenever a therapist *determines,* or pursuant to the standards of the profession *should determine,* that his patient presents a serious danger of violence to another."[33]

The determination of liability hinges upon whether the third party victims were "readily identifiable," and "[w]hether a therapist reasonably should have made these determinations [regarding the seriousness of a threat of violence, and whether disclosure of confidences could prevent the threatened harm] is to be measured against the standard of care in the profession."[34]

In *Hedlund*, a case already discussed, the California Supreme Court made absolutely clear that the malpractice standard of care ought to govern *Tarasoff* actions, by stating that a "negligent failure to diagnose dangerousness in [a] Tarasoff action is as much a basis for liability as is a negligent failure to warn a known victim once such diagnosis has been made."[35]

In *Hedlund*, a mother and child, both injured by a mentally ill patient, alleged a breach of the treating psychologists' duty to them to diagnose the patient and to warn the adult complainant of the danger he posed to her (the injury to her child was viewed as a foreseeable and identifiable injury in the event of an attack on the mother).

Jablonski v. United States[36] upheld a finding that a psychiatrist should have obtained his patient's past medical records from another hospital in order to predict and prevent the patient's murder of a woman friend. The man had been seen in emergency evaluation on two occasions and was apparently a recalcitrant patient. At the trial there had been expert testimony "that under professional standards commonly practiced in the community, [the treating psychiatrist] should have recognized that Jablonski was potentially dangerous,"[37] and should have been made suspicious by the patient's reluctance to discuss his past treatment. If the evaluation had not been negligent the defendants would have known the patient was dangerous, and they would have identified the woman as a forseeable victim.

This case makes clear how the liability of the therapist is greatly expanded when courts using the malpractice standard permit his supposed expertise in evaluating dangerousness, identifying potential victims, and predicting violence to be second-guessed by colleagues testifying as experts about the profession's supposed expertise in these matters. Even when the *Tarasoff* duty is limited to the duty to warn, the malpractice standard allows second-guessing about every act or omission that would have put the therapist in a position to warn. And when the duty to protect is governed by the malpractice standard, liability is opened up even more, amounting, as we shall see, to a version of "strict liability": the therapist is always responsible.

Judges who have fashioned these rules and applied these standards have a powerful answer when they are criticized for placing unfair burdens on psychotherapists. They can say, "If your profession really believes it is impossible to predict violence, then plaintiffs could never obtain credible experts. Apparently there are expert psychotherapists who believe that such predictions are possible and that their accused colleagues are negligent. These experts so testify under oath." We are back to the problem of professional testimony in the courtroom, the ethical and scientific boundaries of such testimony, and the adversarial standard that leads to the phenomenon of experts for hire.

However, it is possible to rationalize the testimony in *Jablonski* as a product of the distinction between expertise in mental status evaluation and in long-term prediction. Experts for the plaintiff were perhaps criticizing the defendants' evaluation. Of course after violence has occurred, a retrospective examination of the psychiatrist's evaluation will often allow the question of negligence to be raised. And do psychotherapists really know what *is* the professional standard of care in evaluating potential violence? Are the clinical procedures clear? Is there evidence they are effective? However one answers these questions, the California Supreme Court was well aware that the malpractice standard would open the doors of the courthouse.

What is more troubling, however, is the Court's pious rhetoric about protecting the public as a justification for placing this burden on psychotherapists. This rhetoric seems even more hypocritical when the police who decided not to confine Poddar were found not to be liable. Can courts claim to be protecting the public when they assign police duties to psychotherapists and absolve the police of those same duties?

The *Tarasoff* decisions are the product of a court that is unwilling to admit the consequences for public safety of the recent general trend, in which it has played a substantial role,[38] toward increasing recognition of the rights of the mentally ill, and the resulting change in civil commitment procedures. The California legislature was in the vanguard of these developments. In passing the Lanterman-Petris-Short Act,[39] it made civil commitment more difficult to initiate and even more difficult to prolong.[40] Indeed, the Poddar case is an example of these new difficulties of initiating commitment. The psychiatrists at the student health facility did not have the authority to confine Poddar on the basis of their own judgment that he was mentally ill and dangerous.

And on the basis of my understanding of common practice in California, I am willing to speculate that an element in the decision of the campus police not to take Poddar to an authorized detention facility was their experience that someone like him under the new laws would be back on the street in a few days, resentful of police intervention.

These sweeping legal reforms mean that society must tolerate greater disturbance in the community and greater risks of harm to the public. Attempts like that of the *Tarasoff* court to avoid these results by exposing therapists to greater liability are self-defeating. Because of its effect on both therapists and patients, a duty to protect third parties will result either in a lower level of safety for society as psychotherapists avoid dangerous patients in order to avoid liability, or, as psychotherapists attempt to carry out their new duty, it will result in futile warnings and increased revolving-door civil commitments.

THE SPECIAL RELATIONSHIP

Even before considering *Tarasoff*'s negative impact on the provision of mental health care, one can see that Fleming and Maximov's analysis of tort law does not provide a legal foundation for their position. They and the court argue that the therapist-patient relationship is sufficiently "special" to justify overriding the usual presumption that there is no duty to control the conduct of a third person so as to prevent him from causing harm to another.

Focusing on cases in which the defendant had control over someone who was dangerous as a result of a "social or mental maladjust-ment,"[41] the authors rely on particular cases in which hospitals have been held liable for suicides or violence against others resulting from negligent control of suicidal or homicidal patients.[42] They admit that the distinguishing factor in the cases in which liability has been found is that the defendant had a *right to control* in addition to *de facto control* over the conduct of another, but suggest that such a right should not be necessary for the imposition of a duty to protect third parties.

Turning to other jurisdictions for support, Fleming and Maximov cite a case in which a hospital was held liable for failure to render emergency care[43] and one in which a state mental hospital was held liable for an assault by a patient whom it negligently failed to admit although the clinical director on standby was aware of his homicidal state.[44] "[A]n even more compelling duty to protect a foreseeable victim would arise *a fortiori*," they assert, "once the culprit had actually been admitted for therapy and a doctor-patient relationship established."[45]

This rationale misconceives both the ground for the imposition of the duty in the cases the authors cite and the nature of the doctor-patient relationship. The language "admitted for therapy" is particularly misleading in its implications about the nature of the therapeutic relationship. Entering a therapist's office is not the the same as being admitted to a mental hospital or being brought to the emergency room.

The imposition of the duty in the cases cited as precedents was based on the fact that the relationship was one of control or, in one case,[46] on the fact that there was a duty on the part of a hospital to establish control. (The director of the hospital had been told that the patient was homicidal. The patient sat in the waiting room for hours and then got up and left.)

The authors simply ignore the fact that the therapist seeing an outpatient in a clinic or office has no control over the patient. Indeed, lack of control is the end sought by much recent mental health case law and legislation, an end Fleming and Maximov strongly support. Moreover, as subsequent cases have made clear, not even the special features of the psychotherapeutic relationship are relevant. Any patient seeing any psychotherapist for any purpose is deemed to have a special relationship. A single diagnostic interview is enough to create a special relationship.

This reasoning follows from the law of malpractice, where generally a doctor-patient relationship begins for some purposes as soon as the doctor agrees to see the patient. Such a relationship, however, involves no control and no psychotherapeutic involvement that makes it special in any sense suggested by Fleming and Maximov. The *Tarasoff* decisions never defined psychotherapist and never addressed the question of when a psychotherapeutic relationship exists—when it becomes legally "special." Had Justice Tobriner, the author of the *Tarasoff* decisions, made the attempt, he might have seen how problematic was the argument about the special relationship.

The *Brady* plaintiffs who sued Hinckley's psychiatrist claimed that Doctor Hopper had had the legal power to commit John Hinckley and therefore the right to take control of him. This argument stands Fleming and Maximov's entire thesis on its head, but in certain respects it is much more reasonable. The plaintiffs argued, "if Doctor Hopper had properly performed his professional duties, he would have controlled Hinckley's behavior"[47] and thereby prevented the assassination attempt and the concomitant injuries to the plaintiffs. The *Brady* court cited *Megeff v. Doland*, which stated, "It is fundamental that in order to take charge of a person in such a manner as will create a duty to control his conduct, one must possess the ability to control that person's conduct."[48]

Whether a *Tarasoff* duty should be premised on the psychiatrist's or psychologist's ability to initiate emergency civil commitment is problematic, as we shall see. The logic is that the power to initiate emergency control is what makes the relationship special. But that argument also suggests that the duty in such situations is to exercise that control. To follow that logic would be to embrace a policy encouraging civil commitment, and that result is just what the California court was attempting to avoid.

Putting aside the ability to initiate civil commitment, different settings for therapist-patient relationships—whether a patient is already committed to a mental hospital, is an inpatient or outpatient in a community clinic, has ongoing private therapy, or has only sporadic contact with a therapist—have different implications regarding the therapist's ability to control the patient, and perhaps even to have the capacity to investigate the patient's dangerousness. *Tarasoff* ignored all of these issues by calling the psychotherapist-patient relationship special and analogizing it to control.

A recent Vermont case provides one illustration of what kind of inquiry can be opened up by this unexamined special therapeutic relationship. In *Peck v. The Counseling Service of Addison County, Inc.*,[49] parents of a voluntary outpatient being seen by a mental health worker in a community mental health clinic sued the clinic for negligent failure to warn them of danger posed by their son. The son was being seen in the counseling service by a counselor and not by a psychiatrist or a Ph.D. psychologist. Is this a special relationship sufficient to impose duties?

Presumably there is no question here of any real control by the counselor or the clinic. Who in such a situation should have the duty to warn or protect? The plaintiffs argued that if the counselor had been properly supervised, the danger that their son would commit arson would have been recognized and so there could and would have been a warning. The defendant-appellees contrasted the situation at hand with situations which involve "a real element of physical control because of the institutional setting," arguing that "in no sense did the Counseling Service have the right or ability to control John Peck. . . . "[50]

The lower court's opinion made it clear that the only reason the decision was not for the plaintiff was because Vermont did not have a *Tarasoff* action as yet. Apparently the judge considered a counseling relationship in a clinic to be presumptively a special relationship. With this invitation from the lower court, the case is in the Vermont Supreme Court at this writing. But the case suggests the growing ramifications of *Tarasoff*.

Clinics which have therapists without advanced training and without their own malpractice insurance may create liability for their employers in *Tarasoff*-type cases. The special relationship can be expanded to include any counseling relationship. The Vermont Psychiatric Association, still fighting the duty to warn and locked into the facts of this case, argued in an *amicus* brief in *Peck* that the duty in such cases should be to commit. The counselor, of course, had no special authority to commit. So that argument seems to win this case. But apparently the Association failed to recognize that the duty to commit, if imposed by the Vermont Supreme Court, opens psychiatrists up to much more potential liability than does the duty to warn.

THE *TARASOFF* DUTY: IMPACT ON THE PROVISION OF MENTAL HEALTH SERVICES

Originally the *Tarasoff* decisions were seen by some as problematic because they put the psychotherapist in an ethical dilemma. Should he warn the victim even when that warning might be detrimental to the patient? But that basic dilemma already existed in the American Psychiatric Association's own Principles of Ethics, which allowed psychiatrists to reveal confidences to protect society. *Tarasoff*, however, added the therapist's own interest in avoiding liability to the balance. It also seemed that the duty to warn threatened third parties, which entailed overprediction, would imperil the therapeutic alliance and destroy the patient's expectation of confidentiality, thereby thwarting effective treatment and ultimately reducing public safety.

Many therapists believed that the nature of the illness and treatment of the kind of potentially dangerous person who voluntarily comes to therapy makes the imposition of such a duty particularly destructive. Such a person is typically not a hardened criminal but rather a person whose violence is the product of passion or paranoia.[51] The object of that passion or paranoia is most often a person of intense significance to the patient.[52] Such, of course, was the case with Poddar in the *Tarasoff* case.

When a therapist tries to deal with the patient's potential for violence, he or she must enter into a therapeutic alliance in which feelings are acknowledged at the same time that the impulses to act them out are discouraged. To maintain this attitude of respect for and acceptance of the patient's feelings while discouraging any violent action is often the central task of the therapist. If all goes well, the patient whose feelings are accepted will come to trust the therapist and be able to explore and understand his violent impulses and consider meaningful alternatives to them.[53]

Given the special significance of the potential victim to those whose violence is the product of passion and paranoia, it might be destructive to the tenuous therapeutic alliance for the therapist to inform the patient that he has a legal duty to protect, and perhaps to warn directly, the potential victim. And there might be even more disastrous therapeutic consequences if one warns the person without telling the patient. (I am not speaking here of the acute emergency situation in which a patient tells his therapist he is going home to kill his family—an emergency that requires immediate intervention by the therapist no matter what the consequences for the therapeutic relationship.) Later commentators would downplay these concerns, as we shall see.

THE MERITS OF THE DUTY TO WARN

Although Fleming and Maximov fail to recognize the possibly destructive consequences for the therapeutic relationship of a duty to disclose confidential information to threatened parties, they acknowledge that such a duty imposes on the therapist an obligation to advise his patients of its existence before beginning treatment.[54] The potentially violent patient is therefore to be greeted with a *Miranda*-type warning as he begins therapy so he can elect to conceal any violent intentions if he believes it to be in his best interest.

Fleming and Maximov cite Perls and Rogers for the proposition that this is no problem because facts are irrelevant to effective therapy, and therefore the withholding of such information will not adversely affect therapy. This conclusion is absurd, and misinterprets and misunderstands Perls and Rogers. These therapists do not contend that facts are irrelevant to effective therapy, but rather focus on the states of feeling and attitudes accompanying the patient's presentation of facts.[55]

Placing constraints on the patient's recitation of facts cuts off the flow of feelings and attitudes that is central to the therapeutic endeavors of the practitioner of Perls' and Rogers' type of psychotherapy. Indeed, Carl Rogers is best known for his emphasis on establishing an accepting therapeutic attitude.[56] Nothing could be more alien to his approach to treatment than a Miranda-type warning.

Fleming and Maximov characterize as unsubstantiated the claim that patients in general, and dangerous patients in particular, will be alienated from therapy by a Miranda-type warning by the psychotherapist of his duty to breach therapeutic confidences in order to protect third parties. It is true, as they note,[57] that such consequences have not been demonstrated in an empirical study. But it is also true to my knowledge that no one has shown in any empirical study that confidentiality between lawyer and client is essential to good legal services. Nonetheless, lawyers are convinced of its necessity on the basis of their professional tradition and their own clinical experience.

In the absence of a reliable empirical study, a judgment based on clinical experience is obviously preferable to a judgment that contradicts such experience. Although the argument for the least restrictive alternative may be powerful and convincing as it has been applied to civil commitment cases in which the commitment was intended only to help the patient,[58] it is less convincing as a justification for the duty to warn.

The argument that the duty to warn may impair therapy has been rejected by some psychotherapists, particularly those who believe that the one-to-one model of psychotherapy is outmoded as a rigid framework.[59] But even some psychotherapists who practice one-to-one therapy have rejected these arguments, claiming that the duty to warn introduces a reality which permits therapist and patient to address in a helpful way the possibility of violence. Indeed, in some quarters the duty to warn has been embraced as a therapeutic advantage. Such practitioners suggest that even the Miranda-type warnings should be thought of as a useful part of the therapeutic contract.[60]

But even if Miranda-type warnings about the therapist's duty to warn had no adverse impact on therapy, the question that has always puzzled me is what value does a warning have for a victim? Imagine a therapist who, following Fleming and Maximov's balancing test, calls a victim and reports that a patient intends violence to them. What can the victim do? Go into hiding? Call the police?

I have often been consulted over the years by persons threatened by mentally ill people who have delivered their own warnings. It turns out that there is very little these "victims" can do to protect themselves. The police will deal with acute incidents, but if the situation continues and becomes chronic, the police tend to put it on the back burner. The potential victim may be legally entitled to a warning, but the value of that warning is another matter. The arguments and counterarguments are difficult to assess. At least, however, it is reasonable to conclude that the duty to warn is not as unmitigated a disaster for the enterprise of psychotherapy as it once seemed to critics like myself.

Psychotherapists who are proponents of the duty to warn believe that it helps them to test the seriousness of the patient's violent intentions and it shows the patient that his violent intentions are being taken seriously. Patients, they say, are even appreciative that the therapist is concerned enough to give the victim a warning. These descriptions of the therapeutic use of the duty to warn suggest to me, however, that the therapist has actually decided there is no acute emergency: he or she is still in the process of managing a patient whose violence he or she believes can be controlled.

But even if one agrees that the duty to warn can be used in this way and made a positive therapeutic parameter in an ongoing therapeutic relationship when there is a foreseeable victim who can be warned, *Tarasoff*'s legal progeny have now gone beyond that scenario. *Jablonski* involved psychiatrists who were doing an initial evaluation of a patient. They had no ongoing relationship and no therapeutic alliance. Furthermore, there was even good evidence that the victim in that case had known that the killer was dangerous (he had assaulted her mother). In fact, she had been warned by others, if not by the psychiatrists involved.

The legal issue no longer is limited to the duty to warn when one has an ongoing therapeutic relationship. *Tarasoff* has expanded the duty to include giving a *Miranda*-type warning and then conducting the kind of immediate expert evaluation that detects dangerousness and allows for identification of possible victims who must be warned or otherwise protected. Therapists must expertly predict violence. *Tarasoff* assumes and requires instant expertise in evaluating and predicting violence.

If the duty to warn is less problematic to the ongoing enterprise of therapy than it once seemed to be, it is also true that the law of *Tarasoff* has moved on and demands more. The greater demands come from both the further implications of the duty to protect and from imposing the professional standard of care. The therapist's prediction of dangerousness is to be examined by the courts under the ordinary malpractice criterion of "conformity to standards of the profession."[61] One can only wonder what it means to apply this standard to skills which do not exist. As Justice Mosk noted, dependence on such standards "will take us from the world of reality into the wonderland of clairvoyance."[62]

If in law the malpractice standard creates more liability in a *Tarasoff* case than the ordinary negligence standard does, there exists an even broader standard for governing liability, that of strict liability. In effect, this broader standard means that the psychotherapist will be liable whenever violence by a patient occurs. *Davis v. Lhim*[63] is a Michigan case which seems to point in that direction. A voluntary patient admitted to a state mental hospital was subsequently released at his own request. There was no evidence that he was considered dangerous either at the time of his admission or at the time of his discharge. Two months after his release he got into a struggle with his mother, who was trying to keep him from firing a shotgun. It is unclear whether he was trying to commit suicide or had some other intention, but the struggle ended with him killing his mother.

If psychiatrists can expertly evaluate immediate potential for violence, such expertise is clearly irrelevant to a killing that happened two months after discharge. There had been no history of violence before or after the hospitalization; thus there was no past behavior on which to base predictions of future behavior. There had been no threats to the mother which would identify her as a forseeable victim. No previous psychiatrist had considered the one-time patient dangerous. The only evidence remotely relevant to *Tarasoff* duties was found in the patient's medical record from an emergency room where he was seen two years before his psychiatric hospitalization. A note in that record said he had "pace[d] the floor and act[ed] strangely and [kept] threaten-ing his mother for money."[64]

That emergency room note and an expert witness who said the son was "violent prone" was apparently sufficient for a court to determine that the mother was an identifiable victim. The psychiatrists therefore should have warned her, and the warning would have mattered. The psychiatrists were therefore negligent. One is reminded of, "for want of a nail, the shoe was lost; for want of a shoe, the horse was lost; for want of a horse, the rider was lost. . . . " How are psychotherapists supposed to behave responsibly after such expansive *Tarasoff* holdings? How will those psychotherapists who have tried to work with the duty to warn solve these new obligations?

Although the requirements of *Tarasoff,* as expanded, are without meaningful guidance for the psychotherapy profession, their practical

consequences are obvious: the door is open to lawsuits claiming negligent failure to predict dangerousness and to protect the public. Psychotherapists have always been reluctant to treat dangerous patients. Not
only must therapists deal with their own personal distress and fearful
reactions as they become involved in the patient's violent predilections,
but also those who are both mentally ill and dangerous are, because of
the nature of their psychopathology, notoriously difficult to treat.[65]

The new legal constraints imposed by *Tarasoff* and its progeny
may well make effective treatment more difficult to obtain as therapists
worry about their own civil liabilities as well as all of these problems.
Physicians everywhere have become wary of treating the type of
patients who generate malpractice claims. Techniques for avoidance
include refusal to accept the patient and referral to public clinics or to
other specialists. Patients who are bounced around in this way often lose
whatever motivation for treatment they may have. One can only assume
that this, with increasing frequency, will be the experience of the
potentially dangerous mentally ill person. These people now carry the
stigma of "legal trouble" no matter how hard the therapist tries to fulfill
his obligations.

When these patients do get into therapy, liability will have the
additional consequence of aggravating the inevitable tendency to
overpredict dangerousness. The therapist—aware of the unreliability of
his predictions and the fact that if he fails to protect a third party who is
harmed by his patient, he must submit to the hindsight judgment of
hired experts and a jury (and the possibility of what amounts to a strict
liability standard)—can be expected to err on the side of caution.
Therapists predicting dangerousness to avoid personal liability will be
given greater incentives to issue broadside warnings and to push for
involuntary confinement.

WHAT SHOULD BE THE THERAPIST'S OBLIGATION?

Nothing I have said should suggest that therapists have no moral duty
when third parties are immediately endangered by their patients. Rather
the legal duty that the *Tarasoff* court imposes and which subsequent
courts have expanded will reduce, rather than increase, public safety
because it will diminish the motivation of responsible therapists to be
involved with mentally disturbed and potentially dangerous people.
Even psychiatrists who now embrace the duty to warn as an advantage
in dealing with potentially violent patients cannot be sure that a

warning fulfills their legal obligation. The thumb of personal liability now weighs heavily on the scale of clinical judgment.

If *Tarasoff* as expanded is so counterproductive, what if any legal duties should be placed on psychiatrists dealing with potentially danger-ous patients? Tort case law provides no justification for finding in every therapist-patient contact a basis for a special relationship that creates an exception to the general rule that a person has no duty to protect third parties. However, I see no reason not to find a special relationship and impose a legal duty in situations where a moral duty is clear and the action it requires is readily comprehensible to those who have the duty. The duty I describe and the justifications for it have been adopted by one Federal Court.[66]

When the psychotherapist believes the bus is bearing down on the blind man, a special relationship exists, and psychotherapists should in my view have a legal duty to take some responsible action. The action re-quired is clear and obvious in the bus analogy, although even in this case a shouted warning might startle the blind man, causing him to fall off the curb, or he might be deaf and not hear the warning. No warning is without peril, but at least in such situations the moral and legal duty is clear.

Fleming and Maximov's analysis does not justify finding a special relationship and does not suggest a responsible action. It assumes all therapy is a special relationship and demands that the therapist first make the difficult determination of whether his patient is dangerous, and then weigh and balance various conflicting factors to select the option—such as a warning—that is least harmful to the patient's interests. And the *Tarasoff* line of cases, while ignoring the patients' interests, makes similar unrealistic demands.

I remain unconvinced that psychotherapists can reliably evaluate the immediate violent potential of patients. My own clinical experience is that some patients are much less transparent than others. I cannot see through recalcitrant, uncooperative, and defensive patients who con-ceal their violent inclinations. If, however, the therapist believes that he or she has overcome the problems of evaluation and decides that his or her patient is imminently dangerous and that the public and the patient need protection, the therapist does have a special relationship and a clear moral duty that allows a legal duty to be imposed.

Imposing legal obligations and liability only at the point at which the therapist has formed his or her judgment, rather than according to some indeterminate malpractice standard dependent on the "ordinary exercise" of a nonexistent skill, will avoid the obvious tendency towards overprediction of dangerousness. This approach is consistent with— although not identical to—the position of Justice Mosk, who wrote the court's opinion in *Burnick* and was sensitive to the lack of content of any reference to "standards of the profession" in prediction. He argued in his concurring and dissenting opinion in *Tarasoff II* that only after the therapist had made his prediction of violence could the imposition of any duty be justified.[67]

Making the special relationship and the legal duty dependent on the therapist's actual determination of the patient's dangerousness would of course severely limit the number of instances in which suit could successfully be brought. In the usual case, once the therapist is convinced that a patient is imminently dangerous, he or she will take some action. Usually the therapist will try to commit the patient or contact the police. If these measures are not available because of the situation—if, for example, the patient is on his way to kill his family— then a warning may be essential. But only when the psychotherapist has reached the conclusion that an emergency exists, and then fails to act, would liability be imposed.

These will not be cases of medical negligence; they will either be instances (as Judge Mosk suggested) of ordinary negligence or be instances when the therapist has simply failed to act, in wanton disregard of his or her own judgment. I do not suggest what the therapists' legal duties should be, apart from taking some responsible action to avoid a tragedy. By this standard, there was no cause of action in the original *Tarasoff* case. The therapists acted responsibly to avoid a tragedy, and they should not have been held liable for the failings of the police.

THE POLICE, THE LAWYERS, AND THE COURTS

One final inconsistency of the California Supreme Court's decision remains to be discussed. The most striking change between *Tarasoff I* and *Tarasoff II* was the dismissal of the claim against the police. The defendant therapist informed the police of the danger Poddar presented and attempted to have him committed. It was the police who decided not to continue that attempt or to warn Miss Tarasoff. But it is the police who are charged with the protection of society and to whom psychotherapists, like other citizens, turn when violence threatens. And it is the police who are trained and armed to protect themselves as well as others from violence. It is the police who can send squad cars to a victim's house to warn him or her.

Surely, if the court was looking for a "special relationship" that would enable it to find a party to hold liable for the tragedy of Miss Tarasoff's death, that relationship can more easily be found between the police and the members of society whom it is their professional duty to protect than between the therapist and his or her patient.

There are obvious explanations for the court's refusal to allow a cause of action against the police. The police must constantly deal with the potentially violent. Imposing tort liability on them might fill the state's penal institutions, drain the public treasury, or have other unacceptable consequences. But reasons for not imposing liability on the police are not reasons for ignoring the equally unacceptable consequences of imposing liability on psychotherapists.

The California Supreme Court's concern with the increased risk to society is understandable. But their failure to acknowledge that the increased risk is due in part to legal reform is not. These reforms have been far-reaching (as discussed elsewhere in this book). First, psychiatric diagnosis has been repudiated as a basis for involuntary confinement, and the use of legal standards such as "dangerousness" has been mandated. Second, there has been legal repudiation of psychiatrists' competence to predict dangerousness. Third, the criminal due process model has been imposed, with most states raising the evidentiary standard for commitment to that of proof beyond a reasonable doubt. Many civil libertarians would require that some dangerous act has already occurred. Fleming and Maximov support each of these steps as limits on the "legally coercive" decision-making power of the psychiatrist.

My concern here has not been to argue that this recent trend in civil commitment is misguided, or even to take issue with Fleming and Maximov in their belief that California has not gone far enough in protecting patients. I have done that elsewhere. But if society opts for more legal protection for the allegedly committable and for less involuntary confinement, it cannot expect more public protection. And it cannot make up the difference by imposing unrealistic duties on therapists.

The *Tarasoff* court attempted to present a new tort liability as though it were inspired by a policy analysis whose goal was the protection of the public "[i]n this risk-infested society." This claim is particularly misleading if the decision was based on the arguments of

Fleming and Maximov, as it seemed to be. These authors conceived the duty imposed as the least restrictive action the therapist can take against his potentially violent patient. Implicit in that choice is an acceptance of greater risk to society.

Neither the court nor Fleming and Maximov seem willing to recognize that the tragedy of Tatiana Tarasoff has little to do with negligent psychotherapists. Her death is the price society pays for legal policies and constitutional doctrines designed to protect the rights of "alleged mental patients" like Prosenjit Poddar. The expanded *Tarasoff* doctrine will not lower that price. If Poddar had been confined to a psychiatric facility, he would have been discharged long before Tatiana Tarasoff returned to Berkeley. The reality is that the present mental health system lacks the wisdom to predict, the ability to treat, and the security to protect society against violence. *Tarasoff* and its progeny will not change this reality.

The real problem that *Tarasoff* deals with is society's felt need to compensate the victims of violence whom it can no longer protect. In a "risk infested" society where the legal system cannot protect its citizens, it can at least compensate them. From this perspective the psychotherapist's malpractice insurance becomes the deep pocket for a victims' compensation fund. There is now talk of applying the *Tarasoff* duty to lawyers. One wonders whether the courts will take the same view of their colleagues' malpractice insurance as they have towards psychotherapists. There is no moral reason not to.

REFERENCES

1. Poddar's original conviction for second degree murder was reversed for failure to give adequate jury instructions concerning a defense of diminished capacity. *See People v. Poddar*, 10 Cal. 3d 750, 518 P.2d 342, 111 Cal. Rptr. 910 (1974).

2. Personal communication.

3. 551 P.2d 334, 131 Cal. Rptr. 14 (1976).

4. California's civil commitment procedures are governed by the Lanterman-Petris-Short Act, Cal. Welf. & Inst. Code §§5000-5404.I (West 1972 & Supp. 1976). The statute provides the following:

    [W]hen any person, as a result of mental disorder, is a danger to others . . . a peace officer, member of the attending staff, as defined by regulation, of an evaluation facility designed by the county, or other professional person designated by the county may, upon probable cause, take, or cause to be taken, the person into custody and place him in a facility . . . for 72-hour treatment and evaluation.

    Id. §5150 (West Supp. 1976).

5. Most states permit any licensed physician to initiate emergency confinement. *See* S. Brakel and R. Rock, *The Mentally Disabled and the Law* (University of Chicago Press, 1971), Table 3.2, pp. 72–76.

6. Since the letter to the police in fact survives, it is not even certain that an order to destroy it was given. Brief for Respondent Moore at 168, *Tarasoff I*.

7. *Tarasoff v. Regents of University of Cal.*, 108 Cal. Rptr. 878 (Ct. App. 1973), vacated and remanded, 529 P.2d 553, 118 Cal. Rptr. 129 (1974).

8. Cal. Welf. & Inst. Code §5150 (West Supp. 1976).

9. *Tarasoff v. Regents of University of Cal.*, 529 P.2d 553, 118 Cal. Rptr. 129 (1974).

10. 13 Cal.3d 205 (1974).

11. Fleming and Maximov, The Patient or His Victim: The Therapist's Dilemma, *California Law Review*, Vol. 62, p. 1025 (1974). Fleming is a Professor of Law at the University of California, Berkeley, where Maximov was a student at the time the article was written.

12. *See generally* T. Szasz, *The Manufacture of Madness* (Harper & Row, 1970).

13. Fleming, *op. cit.*, p. 1046.

14. *Ibid.*, p. 1065.

15. 551 P.2d 334, 347-48; 131 Cal. Rptr. 14, 27–28.

16. 551 P.2d 334, 346-47; 131 Cal. Rptr. 14, 26–27.

17. Livermore, Malmquist, and Meehl, On the Justifications for Civil Commitment, *University of Pennsylvania Law Review*, Vol. 19, p. 84 (1968). *See also* Stone, *Mental Health and Law: A System in Transition* (National Institute of Mental Health, 1975), pp. 25–40.

18. 551 P.2d 334, 345, 131 Cal. Rptr. 14, 25 (quoting *Bardessono v. Michels*, 3 Cal. 3d 780, 788; 478 P.2d 480, 484; 91 Cal. Rptr. 760, 764 (1970)).

19. Since the primary cause of overprediction is the low base rate of violent behavior among the mentally ill, even the therapist who is usually accurate in his predictions will face essentially the same problem as his less accurate colleagues.

20. See 551 P.2d 334, 346, 347, and n.14, 131 Cal. Rptr. 14, 26, 27, n.14.

21. 83 Daily Journal DAR 2832, L.A. 31676, Super. Ct. No. 345227.

22. *People v. Burnick*, 121 Cal. Rptr. 488, 535 P.2d 352 (1975).

23. *See* American Bar Association Standing Committee on Association Standards for Criminal Justice, *First Tentative Draft, Criminal Justice Mental Health Standards*, Standard 7-3.9(b) (1983).

24. *Landeros v. Flood*, 17 Cal.3d 399, 408 (1976).

25. *Hedlund*, 83 Daily Journal DAR 2832, 2834 (Mosk, J., dissenting).

26. Appelbaum, Tarasoff: An update, *Hospital and Community Psychiatry*, Vol. 32, pp. 14–15 (1981).

27. *Brady v. Hopper*, No. 83-JM-451, (D.Colo., 9/14/83).

28. *Ibid.*, p. 8.

29. *Ibid.*

30. *Ibid.*

31. 102 Cal. App. 3d 594, 162 Cal. Rptr. 724.

32. 102 Cal. App. 3d 594, 594.

33. *Ibid.*, p. 599.

34. *Ibid.*, p. 605.

35. 83 Daily Journal DAR 2832, 2833.

36. 712 F.2d 391 (1983).

37. *Ibid.*, p. 393.

38. *See, e.g., Thorn v. Superior Court*, 1 Cal. 3d 666, 464, P.2d 56, 83 Cal. Rptr. 600 (1970); *In re Lambert*, 134 Cal. 626, 66 P. 851 (1901).

39. Cal. Welf. & Inst. Code §§5000-5404.1 (West 1972 & Supp. 1976).

40. *See* Cal. Welf. & Inst. Code §§5150 (West Supp. 1976); *see also* Stone, *supra* note 17, at 60–65.

41. Fleming, *op. cit.*, at 1028 (quoting Harper & Kime, The Duty to Control the Conduct of Another, *Yale Law Journal*, Vol. 43, pp. 886, 898 [1934]).

42. *See, e.g., Merchants Nat'l Bank & Trust Co. v. United States*, 272 F. Supp. 409 (D.N.D. 1967)(homicide); *Meier v. Ross Gen. Hosp.*, 69 Cal. 2d 420, 445 P.2d 519, 71 Cal. Rptr. 903 (1968)(suicide).

43. *Wilmington Gen. Hosp. v. Manlove*, 54 Del. 15, 174 A.2d 135 (1961).

44. *Greenberg v. Barbour*, 322 F.Supp. 745 (E.D.Pa. 1971).

45. Fleming, *supra* note 15, at 1030 (emphasis added).

46. *Greenberg v. Barbour*, 322 F.Supp. 745 (E.D.Pa. 1971).

47. *Brady v. Hopper, op. cit.*, p. 4.

48. 123 Cal. App. 3d 251, 176 Cal. Rptr. 467 (1981), cited in *Brady v. Hopper, Ibid.*

49. Vermont Supreme Court Docket No. 5114–80Ac.

50. Brief of Defendant-Appellee in the Supreme Court of the State of Vermont, Docket No. 83-062, p. 43.

51. See Lion, Bach-y-Rita, and Ervin, Violent Patients in the Emergency Room, *American Journal of Psychiatry*, Vol. 125, p. 1706 (1969).

52. *See* American Psychiatric Association, *Task Force Report 8, Clinical Aspects of the Violent Individual*, pp. 7–9, 28 (1974).

53. *See generally* J. Lion, *Evaluation and Management of the Violent Patient* (Charles C Thomas, 1972).

54. Fleming, *op. cit.*, p. 1056–1060.

55. *See, e.g.*, C. R. Rogers, *Client-Centered Therapy* (Houghton-Mifflin, 1951); F. R. Perls, *Gestalt Therapy Verbatim* (Bantam Books, 1979).

56. *See, e.g.*, Rogers, *Ibid.*, pp. 19–64.

57. *See* Fleming, *op. cit.*, p. 1039.

58. *See, e.g., Lake v. Cameron*, 364 F.2d 657, 660 (D.C. Cir. 1966).

59. *See* D. B. Wexler, *Mental Health Law: Major Issues* (Plenum Press, 1981).

60. J. C. Beck, When the Patient Threatens Violence: An Empirical Study of Clinical Practice after Tarasoff, *Bulletin of the American Academy of Psychiatry and Law*, Vol. 10, pp. 189–201 (1982).

61. *Tarasoff II*, 551 P.2d at 354, 131 Cal. Rptr. at 34 (Mosk, J., concurring and dissenting).

62. *Ibid.*

63. *Davis v. Lhim*, No. 59284 (Mich. Ct. App., March 21, 1983).

64. *See* discussion by Appelbaum, *Hospital and Community Psychiatry*, Vol. 35, pp. 13–14 (1984).

65. *See* Stone, *op. cit.* note 23, pp. 36–37.

66. *Hasenei v. U.S.*, 541 F.Supp. 999 (1982).

67. *Burnick, op. cit.*

VIII

Sexual Exploitation of Patients in Psychotherapy

TWENTY YEARS AGO FEMALE PATIENTS who claimed that they had been sexually exploited by their psychotherapists were apt to be written off as having psychotic transferences. The presumption, derived from psychodynamic theories, that these reports represented hysterical wish-fulfilling fantasies, was applied even to victims of rape and incest.[1] Today, when there are laws about sexual harassment,[2] when psychiatry has recognized the importance of rape and incest trauma and the frequency of such victimization of women,[3] and when the sexual exploitation of psychotherapy patients has been convincingly documented, our former views seem shocking and inexcusable. The Women's Movement is largely responsible for this rude awakening and for the demystification of sexual crimes, sexual exploitation, and sexual harassment.

However, for the psychotherapy establishment a major confrontation with this reality came from Masters and Johnson. At the peak of their influence as the most important sexologists since Kinsey, Masters and Johnson published a book on sex therapy.[4] They reported that a significant percentage of the women who came to their clinic for sexual therapy had been sexually exploited by their previous therapists. Among

these therapists were obstetricians, gynecologists, psychiatrists, psychologists, and social workers, as well as family and pastoral counselors.
None of the helping professions, including the ministry, was free of the
scandal.

Questionnaire surveys, though not without methodological im-
perfections, seemed to confirm Masters and Johnson's impression that
sexual exploitation of women in psychotherapy has been more common
than anyone had realized.[5] Responsible professionals began to discuss
the problem, and the media gave massive publicity to it.[6] The legal and
ethical aspects of sexual exploitation became very important for the
psychotherapy establishment. Most, though not all, of the legal and
ethical complaints involved male therapists sexually exploiting female
patients. I wrote about this problem and the possible avenues of redress
in 1975[7] and have since been consulted by a number of female patients
seeking advice about how to proceed in such situations, as well as by
psychiatrists trying to deal with ethical complaints and the conflicts and
difficulties involved in passing judgment on a colleague. The sample is
by no means large, but what I have learned is chastening.

First, my impression is that none of the women who have
consulted me were fabricating. If once on the basis of my professional
training I presumed that such complaints were false, I now presume that
they are true. There are those who criticize this view, both because the
accused therapist is himself so vulnerable to a false claim, and because it
seems to fly in the face of the traditional legal presumption of innocence.
But as much as I sympathize with the vulnerability of a person wrongly
accused, I am not a court. I do not have the power of government
authority which is held in check by the presumption of innocence. I am
describing my clinical impression and how it has changed. The presumption of innocence is irrelevant to that impression. Indeed, for me to
presume that the therapist is innocent requires me to assume that the
patient is fabricating. And to assume that in my experience is a matter of
the profession's own wish-fulfilling fantasy.

Second, no amount of training or personal psychoanalysis seems to
confer immunity on therapists; nor does position or status at the top or
the bottom of the psychotherapy establishment. Third, if sexual exploitation is traumatic to the patient, so are the attempts to obtain redress.
One patient described it to me: "I felt like I was treated as a criminal,
that they did not take my complaint seriously, and that they wanted me
to go away and not bother them. The therapist's rights were carefully
protected . . . I had no rights, respect, or courtesy." Fourth, although
principles of ethics require us to expose sexually exploitive colleagues,

those who do are apt to be reminded of the maxim, "no good deed goes unpunished." One psychiatrist describing his efforts to assist a woman in her complaint told me that he was made to feel that he was the one behaving unethically. These situations are filled with ambivalence for everyone involved, including the victims, the victimizers, and those who sit in judgment. The scandal created by the publicity given to this subject has hurt the profession, and particularly male psychotherapists.

Psychotherapists of course are schooled in being nonjudgmental, and understandably a typical impulse is to solve the problem by getting the offending therapist into treatment or supervision. Sometimes this impulse is the right solution, but like all therapeutic solutions of moral problems, it has its limitations.

Finally, although sexual exploitation in psychotherapy continues, there is reason to hope that it is diminishing, partly because the public scandal has had a useful educational impact on patients and therapists alike. However, even if this optimistic impression is correct, for the decade of the 1980s the fallout will probably continue because of the typical delay between such incidents and subsequent complaints, and then between the complaints and some appropriate resolution.

Although, as mentioned, the understandable response of the psychotherapy profession is that the therapist should be helped, Masters and Johnson in an address to the American Psychiatric Association took the punitive point of view. They declared:

> We feel that when sexual seduction of patients can be firmly established by due legal process, regardless of whether the seduction was initiated by the patient or the therapist, the therapist should initially be sued for rape rather than malpractice, i.e., the legal process should be criminal rather than civil. Few psychotherapists would be willing to appear in court on behalf of a colleague and testify that the sexually dysfunctional patient's facility for decision making could be considered normally objective when he or she accepts sexual submission after developing extreme emotional dependence on the therapist.[8]

Although one can sympathize with their moral indignation and their demand for punishment, it is by no means clear that criminal prosecution for rape is the most sensible way to proceed. The realities involved in the phrase "can be firmly established by due legal process" turn out to be much more complicated and difficult than the authors might imagine.

In the first place, Masters and Johnson were addressing the case of female patients who were seeking sex therapy. However, sexual exploitation by psychotherapists has not been confined to such patients. Second, they assume that the patient has developed "extreme emotional

dependence"; presumably this is their way of describing the transference relationship. They assume on this basis that the patient should be
considered incompetent to make a decision about engaging in sex. These
are all problematic legal assumptions and they are complicated by the
fact that whether sex even took place is a matter of one person's word
against another's. There often will be no corroborating evidence of this
kind of exploitative rape—that is, no witnesses, physical injury, or other
objective evidence. And in the criminal courts due process requires that
proof of guilt be beyond a reasonable doubt.

Although there is considerable legal debate about the definition of
rape, the trend is to think of rape as a crime of violence.[9] Although rape
can occur in the psychotherapist's office and although it may be
appropriate to make all sexual exploitation of patients a crime, it is by no
means clear that all sexual exploitation should be classed as rape, or that
prosecution for rape is the most expeditious approach.

These problems can be minimized to some extent by a different
approach. That is, one can assume that the psychotherapist has a
fiduciary relationship to the patient. This assumption is in keeping with
both ethical and legal approaches, as we shall see. That a therapist as a fiduciary has a special obligation not to take sexual advantage of a patient
readily fits within this framework. Violations of fiduciary obligations
can be made a crime, not necessarily rape, and they are also relevant to
claims of malpractice. This approach is objective, in the sense that it
does not require inquiry into the patient's transference or her capacity to
consent or her reasons for seeking therapy. Although it does not solve
the corroboration problem, it provides a bright line on the other
questions.

SEEKING REDRESS

There are three possible punitive legal sanctions against a therapist who
has sex with a patient. First, there are the various statutes of the criminal
law, including rape and rape by fraud or coercion. The latter at least
theoretically might be applicable to the situations Masters and Johnson
had in mind. Recently, some states have passed legislation which, in
keeping with the approach outlined above, makes sexual exploitation of
patients a crime which does not require proof of fraud or coercion.[10]
The psychotherapist who has sex with a patient has simply crossed a
bright line, making him a criminal offender though not a rapist.

Second, there are tort actions, including malpractice, in the civil courts. Third, there is revocation of license to practice by a medical board of licensure. Beyond these legal approaches are the ethical sanctions of professional associations, societies, and institutions—sanctions which might potentially be punitive by limiting career opportunities, patient referrals, and staff privileges at various institutional facilities.

A woman seeking redress may be unaware of these various possibilities, as may be the psychotherapist or even the lawyer she turns to for assistance. It is therefore appropriate to detail these possibilities and their consequences. Although today a psychotherapist who sexually exploits a patient may face ethical sanctions, loss of license, a civil suit, criminal charges, damage to his professional reputation, and bankruptcy, these punitive possibilities are rarely realized.

CRIMINAL LAW

The criminal courts have been extremely reluctant to adopt Masters and Johnson's suggestion regarding sex between therapists and patients, for reasons already indicated—the usual absence of violence or threats of violence and the presumption that the woman had a choice. Rape charges apparently are rarely brought against psychotherapists. The few reported cases have involved some element of physical coercion or force rather than the kind of psychological coercion Masters and Johnson referred to. In fact, in cases in which psychiatrists have been convicted of rape, their behavior has been egregious by almost any moral or legal standards.

Thus, an East Coast psychiatrist who gave his patients electroconvulsive therapy and/or injections of hypnotic drugs and then had intercourse with them was convicted of rape and served time in prison.[11] Odious practices like this are not confined to psychotherapists. Similar charges have been leveled against physicians, dentists, and others with the means to render patients unconscious. In another reported case, a West Coast psychiatrist who had intercourse with a sixteen-year-old girl who was referred for therapy for promiscuity was prosecuted for and convicted of statutory rape.[12] These extreme and lurid cases, whether or not they involve psychotherapists, do not require courts to consider subjective notions of transference or consent in order to determine whether rape has occurred.

In contrast to these cases, when a legally competent patient is told that sexual intercourse or some other sexual activity is to be administered as therapy and the patient consents, the prevailing judicial opinion is that there is no rape because there has been neither force nor fraud. However, a few states have passed statutes that specifically make such activity punishable as rape. The clearest example is a Michigan statute that defines coercion in rape to include the following: "When the actor engages in the medical treatment or examination of the victim in a manner or for purposes which are medically recognized as unethical or unacceptable."[13] Under this statute sex as therapy could be construed as rape. But none of these criminal statutes seem to apply to some of the most common forms of therapist exploitation of patients, in which the therapist tells the patient that sex is not therapy but uses the transference relationship to induce compliance. Wisconsin, however, has passed a criminal statute that simply makes it a crime for a psychotherapist to engage in sexual activity with a patient.[14]

Unless new criminal statutes like those in Wisconsin are enacted, criminal charges of rape or related sexual offenses against psychotherapists who exploit their patients are a remote possibility. As we shall see, the burdens on a woman attempting to seek redress in the criminal courts whether for rape or some lesser offense are considerable. Although the consequences of such a criminal conviction may be the loss of the therapist's license to practice, it is likely that the criminal sanction will be no more than probation or a suspended sentence except in the most egregious cases.

CIVIL LAW

The civil area involves suits for damages, and particularly malpractice damages. It is in this area that the most important developments have occurred. Six figure damage awards have been handed down against psychiatrists for negligence involving sex with patients.[15] Although there have been scattered instances of claims and significant legal precedents, it was not until 1975, in *Roy v. Hartogs*,[16] that courts began to award substantial damages and clearly recognized that sexual exploitation of patients was malpractice.

Psychodynamically speaking, there is no doubt that transference enters into many relationships: teacher-student, lawyer-client, physician-patient, and so on. However, it is only in psychotherapy that the management of the transference and countertransference is considered a central feature of the treatment. A Florida court dealt with a case on that very issue in 1972. A psychotherapist treating a woman who was a

patient in a psychiatric hospital told his patient that he was going to divorce his wife and wanted to marry her. The court, after hearing expert
testimony about managing the transference and countertransference,
ruled that the psychiatrist had engaged in "conduct below acceptable
psychiatric and medical standards."[17] The husband had sued the
hospital and was allowed to recover the cost of his wife's hospitalization
and treatment.

The decision's legal basis was in the notion of contract, and there
was no allegation of sexual involvement. Allegations of medical malpractice require the party bringing the suit to produce expert testimony
about the professional standard of care and testimony as to how the
allegedly negligent behavior deviated from that standard. The psychiatric experts in this case in effect testified that the professional standard
of care required psychiatrists to manage the countertransference and the
psychiatrist deviated from that standard by acting out his countertransference in an inappropriate profession of love.

This law suit was brought after the patient had committed suicide,
and no doubt the legal proceedings took place under the shadow of that
event. Here was a husband paying a psychiatrist to treat his wife; the
psychiatrist had asked her to marry him, and the treatment had ended in
the patient's suicide.

Husbands have not, however, fared well in court when they have
sued psychiatrists for having sex with their wives. Many states have
passed so-called heart balm statutes[18] that bar civil liability for sexual
activity in the form of seduction, alienation of affections, or criminal
conversation. It is the heart balm act that prevents husbands from
collecting judgments against their wives' therapists. The wife might
bring such a suit but the husband has no cause of action—that is, no
right to sue on his own behalf. The law is less clear about what would
happen were husband and wife in conjoint therapy and the therapist
had sex with the wife. The husband has a doctor-patient relationship of
his own to complain about in such cases.

In one case that was settled out of court, a husband brought suit in
a state that did not have a heart balm statute. His wife, from whom he
was separated, had worked for a sex therapy clinic as a sexual surrogate.
He sued the clinic not for malpractice or medical negligence, but for
being involved in what the law euphemistically calls "criminal conversation," a sexual tort. These "sexual" torts were originally formulated
in terms of interference with the husband's property and sexual interests
in his wife. A husband could therefore sue the *other* man for adultery or,
as it is called in the antiquated tort context, "criminal conversation."

Prosser, in the standard text on torts, explains that recovery was based on "defilement of the marriage bed [and] the blow to family honor."[19]

"Alienation of affections" was a similar kind of tort which involved depriving the husband of his wife's love; it was not necessary for this charge that the wife have committed adultery. The essence of this tort is interference with the wife's attitude towards her husband. Traditionally, in our male-oriented Anglo-American culture, the wife had none of these remedies. But gradually, women were also deemed entitled to bring some of these suits.

Obviously the logic behind these causes of action has lost much of its compelling force. Many legislatures have taken the position that such suits, along with actions for breach of promise to marry, more often serve as instruments of blackmail than as compensation for tortious injury. Legal scholars increasingly have become convinced that money damages do not provide "heart balm." Moreover, there have been such dramatic changes in modern attitudes towards sex, marriage, and divorce that many of these tort actions seem Victorian. Thus, beginning in the 1930s, the so-called heart balm statutes were passed in many jurisdictions. However, in the few jurisdictions that do not have such statutes, husbands might have grounds for suit.

In *Roy v. Hartogs*, Doctor Hartogs' lawyers claimed that the heart balm act meant there could be no basis for a malpractice suit by the patient. That is, they argued, sexual activity (not rape) could not be the basis of a civil suit. However, the court held that the relationship of a psychotherapist to a patient was a "fiduciary relationship" analogous to that between a guardian and his ward. Further, the court stated that "there is a public policy to protect a patient from the deliberate and malicious abuse of power and breach of trust by a psychiatrist when that patient entrusts to him her body and mind."[20]

This judicial decision analogizing the therapist-patient relationship to the guardian-ward relationship not only undercuts the relevance of the heart balm act but also does away with the difficult problem of consent. "Consent obtained under such circumstances is no consent, and should stand for naught."[21] The court's reasoning is similar to that of the new criminal statutes which have already been discussed. The difficult question of whether the patient had the capacity to consent becomes irrelevant. Of course, this reasoning might offend libertarians and it does offend some feminists, because it can be interpreted as a continuing form of male chauvinism in which women, if not considered property, are treated as if they were children who are incompetent to make their own sexual decisions.

Although idealization of the therapist's authority and erotic over-estimation of him are common, the legal analogy to a guardian-ward relationship does not capture the subtleties of transference, nor does it credit the patient-ward as being capable of autonomous choice. Perhaps the best way to understand the court's decision is to see it as reaching for a way to say that the psychotherapist has a duty not to become sexually involved with a patient, even if she maturely consents. Such a decision is fully compatible with the testimony given by Doctor Willard Gaylin in *Roy v. Hartogs*: "there are absolutely no circumstances which permit a psychiatrist to engage in sex with his patient."[22] All such instances constitute malpractice.

However, if one asks why such a duty should be imposed on a psychotherapist, the answer brings us back to the vulnerability of the patient to being coerced by the transference, or the related idea that troubled people are vulnerable when they turn to a therapist for help. But these same considerations often are equally relevant to the physician-patient and the divorce lawyer–client relationship, contexts in which sexual exploitation allegedly is at least as common as it is in psychotherapy. Yet courts have not, for example, allowed patients to sue obstetricians and gynecologists for malpractice when there is also arguably sexual exploitation of the patient based on transference. Although in these instances the moral wrong may be as great as it is when therapists have sexual contact with patients, obstetricians, gynecologists, and lawyers do not hold themselves out as providing a service or a treatment that has as a central feature managing the transference and countertransference. This feature of the therapist's role is a valid justification for the law's singling out psychotherapists.

But there are psychotherapists who reject the whole notion of transference and countertransference, and there are behavior therapists and biological psychiatrists who treat patients in a relatively impersonal manner: in their cases this justification may not apply any more convincingly than it does to other physicians.

Whatever the convincing theoretical justification may be for singling out psychotherapists, the facts alleged in court cases suggest unethical and grossly negligent behavior. For example, in *Roy v. Hartogs* it was alleged that a patient with homosexual concerns and feelings of heterosexual inadequacy was induced to have repeated sex with her psychiatrist during treatment sessions as a form of therapy to overcome these problems. There was in this case, as in all sexual situations which take place in private, the problem of corroborating the patient's testimony. Ordinarily in such cases testimony as to similar conduct by the psychiatrist could be excluded, but the psychiatrist in this case denied having sex with the patient and claimed to be impotent. Therefore, the patient was able to offer the testimony of three other women patients, two of whom reported similar sexual experiences with the psychiatrist and the third who described blatant and inappropriate sexual behavior and attempted seduction by him.

Some of this damaging testimony was stricken from the record as not relevant to the time period during which the psychiatrist claimed impotence. But it is hard to believe the jury ignored it. The psychiatrist claimed that the two patients whose testimony was admissible were both, like the patient who brought suit, suffering from erotomania. The jury, after a lengthy trial, awarded the patient 250,000 dollars in compensatory damages and 100,000 dollars in punitive damages. Obviously, it is no easy matter for jurors to decide what the damages are in such cases. Here there was evidence that the patient's mental health had deteriorated after this treatment. She had been unable to continue her employment and she had been distrustful of other psychotherapists. Finally, she had to be hospitalized in a near catatonic state. However, these large damage awards did not remain in effect.

MALPRACTICE INSURANCE

The reasons for the revocation of the amount of damages are quite complex, and there were other complicating circumstances. First, the therapist's malpractice insurer refused to defend him, leaving the therapist to support three years of litigation on his own. The insurers claimed that sex with a patient was not professional conduct covered by their policy. However, after the damage judgment was awarded, the patient sued the insurance company for the damages and settled for 50,000 dollars, which was one-half of Doctor Hartogs' liability coverage.

A similar case decided years before had held that sexual exploitation was covered by the doctor's liability policy.[23] Hartogs paid for and pursued his own legal appeals of the jury verdict against him, and a subsequent decision in a higher court dismissed the punitive damages of 100,000 dollars and reduced the compensation award to no more than 25,000 dollars. Although Hartogs' insurance company had settled with the patient, it nonetheless refused to compensate Hartogs for his considerable legal expenses. He therefore sued the insurance company. In a decision that suggests rough justice but somewhat incoherent legal reasoning, the court rejected Doctor Hartogs' suit.[24] The results of all of this maneuvering were quite confusing. Psychotherapists could be sued for sexual exploitation as malpractice. The insurer need not defend them but might have to pay damages.

There soon followed a number of law suits in various states alleging malpractice based on sexual exploitation of patients. If psychotherapists had to pay out of pocket for their own legal defense, it was unlikely that they would have enough money left to pay damage awards if found guilty. If such conduct was not malpractice covered by the therapist's policy, then large damage awards would probably be uncollectable. These issues were of considerable concern to the insurers as well as to the therapists against whom complaints were made.

There is an important issue which further complicates these matters. Even if one is prepared to argue that sex with patients is so obviously unethical that it is outside the scope of professional activity that should be indemnified by liability insurance, one cannot say the same about false accusations of sexual activity by a patient. Such accusations might happen to the most scrupulously ethical therapist practicing psychotherapy of a high standard. Whatever one's presumption may be, not every complaint is true; some are fabricated or even malicious. If it is reasonable to assert that there are some such cases, then surely a malpractice policy should at least provide a falsely accused therapist with a legal defense. The American Psychoanalytic Association, not wanting to indemnify sexually exploitative therapists but wishing to protect innocent therapists from false claims, tried to tailor their liability policy to that end. This was easier said than done.

Insurance companies routinely make economic calculations about the cost of a legal defense versus a settlement versus a predicted jury verdict. If the insurance company is responsible only for the cost of the legal defense, then there is an immediate conflict of interest with the therapist whose reputation is at stake and who, if he loses the case, will be personally responsible for the damages. How does the insurance company decide whether the therapist is falsely accused? He may want the best and most expensive legal defense he can get in order to protect his reputation even if he is guilty. Furthermore, if he, not the insurance company, has to pay any settlement, how can the insurance company's lawyer represent him? He has everything to gain and nothing to lose while the insurance company has nothing to gain and everything to lose from the expensive litigation process.

Although there are often conflicts of interest between therapists charged with malpractice and their insurance companies, a policy which provides a legal defense for a doctor who claims to be innocent but then makes the doctor responsible for the damages is particularly precarious. There are a number of ways to cope with these potential conflicts. The policy might, for example, provide a specific amount for legal defenses in such cases. But this and other schemes may be impractical. The American Psychological Association pursued an alternate course. Their insurance policy excludes liability for sexual activity. For this and other reasons their liability premiums are minimal.

Whether the adverse effects of sex between therapist and patient should be compensable by an insurance policy is a debatable question. To some it seems immoral to protect a psychotherapist against the consequences of his immoral actions. But if one believes that patients are harmed by such sexual exploitation, and if the courts do permit suits for malpractice, then the result of eliminating insurance coverage is to make it highly unlikely that victims will be compensated by a bankrupted defendant. Punishing the therapist by not indemnifying him through malpractice insurance also punishes the victims. Coverage according to this view protects the victimized patients; it is a compensation fund to which the community of therapists contributes in the form of higher malpractice premiums.

The American Psychiatric Association has for these and other reasons continued to provide coverage for malpractice involving sexual exploitation. Although the public is more impressed with the scandalous elements of these cases, the American Psychiatric Association appears to be alone among these professional organizations in its concern for the victims who would otherwise go uncompensated. Whether this admirable policy will continue in the face of escalating jury awards to sexually victimized patients and escalating liability premiums remains to be seen.

THE IMPLICATIONS OF *ROY V. HARTOGS*

Despite its important holdings *Hartogs* did not clarify all of the malpractice implications of sex between therapist and patient. There were two lines of defense that this therapist did not assert: (1) that the patient had freely consented to an affair and had known it was not therapy; and (2) that the therapist believed sex between the doctor and patient was therapeutic, and that the patient had been told in advance that sexual activity would be part of the therapy—that is, that she had been given full disclosure before the transference developed. Instead, the therapist insisted that the patient had a psychotic transference. Both of these potential defenses, although ethically unacceptable to the psychotherapy profession, might be tenable defenses in a court of law. The first defense in particular might gain acceptance in court, as intimated by a dissenting judge in *Hartogs*.

Although subsequent courts have had little difficulty in finding psychiatrists negligent and awarding huge damages, there was one dissenting judge in *Hartogs* who was prepared to argue that there was no malpractice and there were no damages. He argued that the civil courts were not the place for dealing with the problems of sex therapy or sex between therapist and patient. As he put it, "Although the plaintiff was suffering from a number of emotional problems, her competency was never placed in issue." Thus he rejected the fiduciary theory, insisting that the patient was legally competent to consent to have intercourse. He went on:

> Is it not fair to infer therefore that she was capable of giving a knowing and meaningful consent? For almost one and a half years while this "meaningful relationship" continued the plaintiff was not heard to complain. Upon the defendant terminating the relationship this law suit evolves.[25]

The judge made it clear that he believed the jury finding that the psychiatrist had had intercourse with his patient and that the psychiatrist "obviously did not help his cause by denying what the jury found to be the fact. . . . Nevertheless, however ill-advised or ill-conceived was the choice of his defense, in my view this did not constitute malpractice." He also stated,

> I neither condone the defendant's reprehensible conduct, nor maintain that it was not violative of his professional ethics and Hippocratic oath. . . . For violation of his Hippocratic oath, if there be any, let him suffer the sanctions of the medical ethics board or other appropriate medical authority.[26]

This proposal to turn the case over to the medical licensing board and the profession for appropriate action was in fact in line with the majority decision, which stated:

> Sex under cloak of treatment is an acceptable and established ground for disciplinary measures taken against physicians either by licensing authorities or professional organizations.[27]

Interestingly enough, the court did not foreclose the matter of whether the psychiatrist should be deprived of his license or sanctioned by his professional organization:

> Whether defendant acted in such manner as to seriously affect his performance as a practitioner in the psychiatric field should be left to these more competent fora. The only thing that the record herein supports is that his prescribed treatment was in negligent disregard of the consequences. For that and that alone he must be held liable.[28]

PROFESSIONAL BOARDS AND ASSOCIATIONS

The licensing boards and professional associations which were consid- ered "the more competent fora" by that court demonstrate an almost total lack of capacity to act. The professional associations have no subpoena power and no expertise in criminal or other evidentiary investigation. They have neither formulated necessary procedures nor employed sufficient legal staff to protect either the due process rights of a doctor charged with some such act or themselves, if the charged doctor sues them.

Indeed, it often happens that, because his or her whole career is at stake, a doctor charged with any ethical complaint hires a lawyer who immediately threatens to sue the professional witness, the society, the association, and its ethics committee for violating the offending doctor's rights. And if the doctor does not follow such legal tactics of harass- ment, he or she will often be motivated to obtain a zealous legal defense. Where will the zealous prosecution come from? The psychotherapy profession lacks the means and often the will to proceed against an unethical colleague.

Ethics committees among professional associations routinely (on request of the therapist's lawyer) postpone action until any pending civil or criminal suit has been resolved. Lengthy court delays are common, and a fresh inquiry by an ethics committee will under these circumstances have to deal with stale evidence and weary protagonists. Even after such a process is complete, the most that a professional association can do is to expel a member—a sanction that has little but symbolic value. In fact, there are cases in which psychotherapists have attempted to resign from an association rather than submit to the ethical inquiry of what is after all a voluntary professional association.

Furthermore, many psychotherapists, as noted previously, react to a colleague's sexual involvement with patients as symptomatic—as an indication that the offender needs treatment and rehabilitation rather than punishment. The extent to which this therapeutic approach will reach was illustrated in a case where a woman who complained about sexual exploitation was induced to enter conjoint therapy with the offender. She and her therapist were being treated in a unique version of couple's therapy.

Thus the failure of professional associations or therapists to respond punitively to offenders in their ranks may to some extent be a product of their members' general therapeutic orientation. But whatever the reasons may be, the results are not often satisfactory to the women who make such an ethical complaint.

Finally, we turn to the licensing boards. The fact that a number of cases exist in which licensing boards have actually revoked licensure for sexual activity of doctors with patients suggests that some power resides in these boards and is being used.[29] However, the licensing boards in each of the states are organized quite differently. Some have a close relationship to the medical society, others do not, and some are impotent bureaucracies reluctant to do anything. Therefore, one cannot expect real consistency across the different jurisdictions. Each jurisidiction has enabling statutes that limit its board's scope of authority.

In one western state, for instance, a physician guilty of the grossest sexual impropriety did not have his license revoked because the only ground was "grossly negligent or ignorant malpractice"; his board had found that he was guilty of "grossly negligent and *immoral* malpractice."[30] Although licensing boards in some states have become much more active and consumer-oriented than this case suggests, they still typically are underfunded by the state legislature and lack the investigatory and legal resources to be as effective as they might be in cases of sexual exploitation.

Although a suit for malpractice seems to be the most powerful approach to punish, discipline, and deter sexual activity between therapist and patient in most cases, even this avenue seems not to provide a fully effective system of control. In the end, in this as in most other things, patients must depend on the decent moral character of those entrusted to treat them. But although none of the avenues for controlling such abuses has proved completely effective, my own impression is that the situation is improving as a result of the greater awareness of both therapists and patients. Still more needs to be done, and the psychotherapy profession, if it has the will to do it, has a special role to play.

THE ROLE OF THE PROFESSION

When a psychotherapist is publicly exposed because of sexually abusive conduct, it often turns out that a substantial number of his or her colleagues acknowledge (usually in confidence) that they had long known of this unethical conduct. Rarely do these colleagues recognize that they may have failed in their own ethical responsibilities. Section two of the American Psychiatric Association's annotated Principles of Medical Ethics[31] directs psychiatrists to "strive to expose those physicians deficient in character and competence." Yet standing in the way of this affirmative ethical duty to expose such physicians is the equally important obligation to protect the confidentiality of patients.

Psychotherapists who are not medically trained face similar ethical dilemmas. Here only the American Medical Association's Principles of Medical Ethics as adapted for psychiatrists and those promulgated by the American Psychoanalytic Association will be considered. Of course it is possible to practice psychiatry, psychoanalysis, and psychotherapy without being a member of any voluntary professional association. Such therapists are answerable for their ethical violations only to the authority that licenses and disciplines them.

There has been great professional opposition against state "snitch laws" that require reporting of deficiencies in a colleague's character and competence to the licensing authority. Of course the profession's principles of ethics already contain "snitch provisions." But such principles of ethics, unlike "snitch laws," can be ignored with absolute impunity. Indeed, many psychotherapists do not even know such provisions exist. There are special problems about reporting the sexual misconduct of colleagues, even when one is aware of one's own ethical obligation.

The psychiatrist has usually heard about his or her colleagues' sexual misconduct from patients in the course of therapy, during consultations, and, perhaps even more often, from other psychiatrists who share such information with the expectation of collegial confidentiality. Often this information is in the form of vague rumors, or even gossip. Rarely is there what could be considered well-documented evidence. Thus on the one hand the psychiatrist typically has only hearsay knowledge of wrongdoing, and on the other hand he or she is bound by section four of the Principles, which requires psychiatrists to "safeguard patient confidences within the constraints of the law."[32] Given these limitations, it is easier to do nothing.

Thus, even when one does recognize the often ignored affirmative duty to "expose" such a colleague, one often feels helpless to do anything. Doing nothing, then, can become the accepted norm of professional behavior, while taking action to expose a colleague can become the deviant exception to this norm. Whatever the reasons for this collective failure to act, in retrospect it creates the appearance of a "conspiracy of silence."

Critics charge that the ethical duty of confidentiality to the patient is used hypocritically to cloak the offending therapist, that psychiatrists are more responsive to the requirements of professional etiquette and to each other than to their professional responsibility to patients, and that the Canons of Ethics protect the profession, and not the patient.[33] It is this kind of criticism that has led to the demand, for example, of legally required reporting of alcoholic physicians. Similar criticisms have been made of other professions, including the legal profession.

Whether or not such criticisms are deserved, it is clear that physicians place a high value on confidentiality—a value that is not limited to patients' confidences. Confidentiality is traditional during the investigation of ethical complaints of doctors.[34] Even after an offending physician has been given a fair hearing, exhausted all appeals, and been sanctioned, that result customarily has remained confidential. Although the impulse to protect a colleague's career and sympathetically to encourage a rehabilitative process is laudable, the possibility of contin-ued abuse of unsuspecting patients is the potential cost of this custom-ary practice. Nowhere in the Canons of Ethics is this potential cost confronted, and nowhere is the psychiatrist given guidance as to how to reconcile the conflicting duties of confidentiality and of exposing unethical colleagues.

Confidentiality has merited special consideration in psychiatry, not only because it is necessary to protect the privacy of patients but also because an expectation of privacy is essential to protect the process of psychotherapy itself—particularly the intimate process of psychoana-lytic therapy. This professional interest has led some psychiatrists to oppose their patients' waivers of confidentiality.[35] Although this oppo-sition has emphasized the patient's interests in confidentiality and the complexities attendant on a fully informed waiver, there is also a professional interest in protecting the therapeutic zone of privacy.[36]

The Canons of Ethics address these legitimate professional con-cerns, but when confidentiality becomes an absolute value—a trump that wins out over all other clinical and ethical considerations—we drastically limit our ability to take responsibility for disciplining our own profession. We fall into a pattern of moral inertia. The annotated

Principles, of course, are not absolute about confidentiality; they make it clear that a psychiatrist may release confidential information with the patient's authorization after "apprising him/her of the connotations of waiving the privilege of privacy."

The American Psychoanalytic Association's Principles of Ethics for Psychoanalysts,[37] in contrast, makes no mention of this alternative. Section six states, "Except as required by law, a psychoanalyst may not reveal the confidences entrusted to him." Although section twelve urges the psychoanalyst to "expose without hesitation, in an ethical fashion and through appropriate channels, illegal or unethical conduct of fellow members of the profession," no guidance is given about such a waiver of confidentiality. How does the psychoanalyst resolve the conflict between section twelve and section six? If we assume that a psychoanalyst has become convinced that a patient has been sexually abused by a colleague, the ethical dilemma is how then to proceed "in an ethical fashion" to expose that colleague's misconduct when that misconduct has become known in a context of confidentiality.

This dilemma is perhaps more common than we generally acknowledge, and it is not just an abstract conflict of two ethical principles. The ethical dilemma is grounded in real clinical problems, which the public and our critics may not fully appreciate. If we examine the ethical dilemma in more detail, the clinical problems will emerge.

It should be clear that there is no ethical dilemma when a patient comes to a psychotherapist and reports that she has been sexually abused by a colleague and asks for assistance in taking some action. The therapist, of course, must make a judgment about the truthfulness of the complaint. Having come to a good faith judgment on that issue, there is no ethical reason standing in the way of helping the patient to assert any ethical or legal claim. A desire not to get involved has no standing as an ethical principle. That is not to deny that such involvement may have costs. In some cases the psychiatrist helping a complaining patient has been treated more harshly by colleagues than by the offending therapist.

THE ETHICAL AND CLINICAL DILEMMA

The ethical and clinical dilemma arises when a patient reports sexual abuse, when the psychiatrist believes her, and the patient for whatever reason seeks no redress. It should be clear to the psychiatrist, if not the psychoanalyst, that the patient can resolve the physician's conflicting ethical duties by waiving confidentiality. At once, however, clinical questions arise. First, should the psychiatrist put this burden on the patient? What is often at issue here is the conviction of the psychoana-lytically oriented psychiatrist that to focus on his or her own ethical dilemma with a patient will disrupt the transference and countertrans-ference, distort the therapeutic process, and give the therapist's con-cerns priority over the patient's treatment. All of this runs counter to traditional psychoanalytically oriented training. Thus, for understand-able and professionally legitimate reasons, psychoanalytically oriented psychiatrists treating a patient who has been sexually abused by a previous therapist may put off raising the ethical problem. Because of that delay, the "decision" to do nothing may become the inevitable result.

More is at stake, however, than technical considerations. In the example of the patient who is believed to have had sex with her previous therapist, the ethically responsible psychiatrist cannot go forward in any useful way without the patient's becoming involved in substantiating the ethical complaint. Such patients often feel guilty, humiliated, and ashamed. Their feelings are not unlike those of a woman who has been subjected to an incestuous relationship with her father. The sexual activity has often taken place in the context of an idealized "father transference," and the woman may not have worked through those transference feelings and what they mean to her. She may be bewildered and uncertain, still in a sense loving the therapist and clinging to the no-tion that the therapist really loved her. These are not easy feelings to sort out.

Just as with incest, once the line of taboo has been crossed, the ordinary categories of human emotion seem blurred and confused. Even if the patient now condemns her therapist-seducer, there is the problem of what kind of and how much punishment she wants to exact and how she feels about making this private matter—including her own sexual activities—public.

Those of us who, on the one hand, have traditional training in psychoanalytic therapy and, on the other hand, are trying to help a patient cope with all of these conflicting emotions are understandably hesitant to push the ethical problem. Furthermore, there can be no doubt that pursuing any kind of ethical or legal complaint will involve the patient in a major real-life commitment. Her credibility may be challenged, and she must endure in the face of adversarial confrontation and procedural delay in order to accomplish anything.

All this must be clearly explained to the patient if she is to make a knowing waiver of confidentiality. Clearly much more is at stake for the patient than for the psychiatrist who is impelled to make an ethical complaint. And, as indicated, the psychiatrist runs the risk of being labeled "judgmental" or a "troublemaker" by some colleagues.

Some patients, of course, will refuse to waive confidentiality even when the psychiatrist does present the ethical issue. How much then should the therapist press the patient and try to convince her that she should waive confidentiality and join the psychiatrist in taking this burdensome step? Some psychiatrists, including even some psychoan-alysts, now believe that it is therapeutically important for sexually abused women to act. The real world confrontation is considered a crucial therapeutic parameter for such a woman to work through in order to master the trauma of this sort of experience.

These therapists see no conflict between clinical and ethical objectives. Rather, they would claim the patient's direct involvement is central to the therapeutic alliance and to a beneficial outcome. They would minimize all of the therapeutic reasons for caution and neutrality described above. Of course, they also recognize that the patient will need considerable emotional support and are prepared to supply it, just as they would with a rape victim.[38] They would argue that the failure to take such action limits the value of any insight therapy, including psychoanalysis.

A POSSIBLE SOLUTION

There is insufficient evidence to choose between these two clinical approaches on empirical grounds. A great deal seems to depend on the values of the therapist. But it is quite clear that traditional approaches may lead to an aggregate failure of ethical responsibility. Ingenious psychoanalytically oriented clinicians have devised sensible procedures to balance these seemingly contradictory approaches.

The therapist-administrator split,[39] whatever its limitations, may be a technical procedure that is particularly applicable in these situa-tions. The therapist who is convinced that a patient has been victimized can suggest to the patient that they both or that the patient alone discuss the situation with a consultant (the administrator). If the patient agrees, thereafter the consultant would assume responsibility for ensuring a knowing waiver of confidentiality. The patient and consul-tant can press appropriate ethical and legal remedies, while the therapist and patient can remain in a traditional therapeutic relationship if that seems desirable.

This step of consultation will not guarantee that an ethical or legal complaint is made; the patient may still decide in favor of privacy and confidentiality. Even more commonly, the patient may remain ambivalent, hurt, and angry but may not want to harm the career or even the marriage of the unethical psychiatrist. The consultation may serve only as an abreaction to an authority figure.

Nonetheless, enlisting a consultant removes some of the traditional inertia. It allows someone who is selected as a consultant because he or she is knowledgeable and skilled about legal and ethical procedures to discuss the matter realistically with the patient. Such consultants could be designated by local psychoanalytic societies and by district branches of the American Psychiatric Association and American Psychological Association.

To use such consultants would be an ethically responsible step for the therapist to take that would violate no ethical principle. Indeed, section nine of the the American Psychoanalytic Association's Principles[40] and section five of the American Psychiatric Association's annotated Principles[41] encourage consultation, although neither explicitly recognizes that consultation should be used for ethical problems of this nature.

Unless convinced that it is contrary to the patient's best interest, the consultant should feel free to encourage the patient to participate in some real-world action (ethical, disciplinary, or legal) against the unethical psychiatrist and should offer to assist in that action.

The consultant should be influenced in this judgment by the circumstances of the sexual abuse and should be particularly concerned when it seems likely that other patients have been abused. Based on my own experience, there seems to be a typology of psychotherapists who sexually abuse patients. First, there is the middle-aged depressed psychotherapist with problems in his own marriage, who becomes involved with a younger woman patient.

Although typically the therapist exploits a positive transference, that exploitation does not involve seduction by charm or malicious exploitation. Rather, the therapist tells the patient his troubles. Often there is talk of divorce and of marrying the patient. It is a scenario not confined to the psychotherapist's office.

Second, there is the psychotherapist who has a bad character in the old fashioned sense. His sexual involvement with patients is only one aspect of his exploitation of his position and the opportunities presented for self-interested gratification. He is manipulative and sociopathic, in his sexual involvements as in other things.

Third, there is the psychotherapist who has some perverse sexual fixation. These perverse impulses are repeatedly acted out on patients. This group would include therapists who have sex with patients they have rendered unconscious. In these cases there is no exploitation of the transference; it is an exploitation of the therapeutic situation.

Fourth, there is the psychotherapist who is sexually "liberated" and who believes that sexual liberation includes sex with patients. He may be more or less public about his sexual ideology. But he uses his position as a psychotherapist to actualize it.

Fifth, there is the psychotherapist who grandiosely loves his female patients and who wants to be loved by them, particularly if they are young and attractive. He wants the intimacy of the therapy to be real. Often he begins by hugging and kissing his patients, but he does not stop there. He, unlike the depressed type, is charming, expansive, and aggressively seductive.

Sixth, there is the psychotherapist who is withdrawn, introverted, uncomfortable with human intimacy. When confronted with a patient who has an intense positive and sexualized transference, he succumbs. In a sense he believes that he has been seduced, but he feels very guilty nonetheless and is quite apt to confess.

As this typology suggests, many psychotherapists become sexually involved with more than one patient. Typology, however, is not enough of an explanation for the widespread sexual exploitation which in my opinion peaked during the decade of the 1970s. Psychotherapy has always been an extremely intimate human experience. The intimacy, moreover, is often erotic in tone rather than platonic.

It seems that sexual liberation in the wider society found its way into the psychotherapist's office and undermined the sense of professional probity. The combination of the social influence of sexual liberation, the intimacy of psychotherapy and the personality of the therapist and patient are all part of the story that would explain the pattern of sexual exploitation of patients. And exploitation it is when a therapist takes advantage of the psychotherapeutic relationship to pursue his sexual gratification.

There are therapists and patients who fall in love. The appropriate ethical behavior under such circumstances is to terminate the therapy and refer the patient to another therapist, informing him or her of the love. The new therapist can help the patient sort out love and idealized transference. When that has happened, a nonprofessional relationship might begin if both parties are still interested.

The typology outlined above can be helpful as a framework for understanding sexual exploitation and making judgments about how to proceed. It can be very important to discuss with the patient whether she believes the therapist is sexually involved with other patients.

If, for whatever reason, the patient does not want to seek redress, there are several less drastic measures a consultant might take. For example, with the patient's consent he or she might notify the offending psychiatrist to seek treatment if that seems appropriate, and warn him about the possible consequences of continued sexual abuses. The offending psychiatrist will at least be on notice that a consultation has taken place and that a concerned and knowledgeable colleague has become involved.

This procedure by no means resolves all problems, but it is preferable to the appearance of moral inertia and a conspiracy of silence. The use of a consultant in this role will not be achieved without complications. The problem of split transference, with the patient playing off one psychiatrist against the other, may occur.

The pursuit of ethical or legal redress may undermine the significance of therapy and the therapeutic alliance. If the patient is married or has close relatives, either the consultant or the therapist will have to deal with their involvement. If legal redress is sought (and based on the analysis in this essay a malpractice suit is usually the most effective redress), the lawyer-client relationship may add further complications. But a sensitive lawyer rapidly takes over the responsibilities of the consultant and encourages the patient's therapeutic relationship with her psychiatrist. The consultant of course should not be a member of any ethics committee that sits in judgment; he or she has already reached a conclusion on the matter.

The vast majority of psychotherapists are ethical and competent. They are deeply troubled by the unethical conduct of the very few who sexually abuse and mistreat patients and discredit the profession. We may feel that these offending colleagues need treatment rather than punishment, but all too often we take no action at all because of our conflicting ethical responsibilities. We owe it to ourselves and our patients to confront publicly the conflicting ethical responsibilities we experience privately. Like our patients, once we openly identify our problems, perhaps we can begin to find more effective ways to deal with them responsibly.

REFERENCES

1. H. Deutch, *The Psychology of Women* (Grune & Stratton, 1945). See especially discussion of rape fantasies in Vol. 1, p. 256.

2. *See, e.g.*, Wisc. General Laws, §111.32 (framing sexual harassment in terms of employment discrimination); Minn. General Laws Annotated, Chs. 609.341 *et seq.*

3. A commonly accepted statistic holds that one out of every three women will be a rape victim over the course of her lifetime. Dickes and Fleming report a study demonstrating that one out of every twenty women is at risk of being raped each year in New Orleans, a representative large urban city. *See* "Sexuality in General Medical Practice," in R. C. Simons and H. Pardes, eds., *Understanding Human Behavior in Heath and Illness*, 2d ed. (Williams & Wilkins, 1981), p. 327.

   Statistics regarding the incidence of incest are less readily available for many reasons. Incest is not one of the FBI's "index crimes," and tends also to be excluded from state-level compilations of crime statistics. It has been estimated that there are somewhere between 40,000 and a quarter of a million cases of incest each year in the United States.

4. W. H. Masters and V. E. Johnson, *Human Sexual Inadequacy* (Little, Brown, 1970).

5. *See, e.g.*, Ethics and the Sensual Psychologist, *Science News*, Vol. 112, No. 19, p. 293 (1977); J. Edelweich, A. Brodsky, *Sexual Dilemmas for the Helping Professional* (Bruner-Mazel, 1982); H. Kardener, Sex and the Physician/Patient Relationship, *American Journal of Psychiatry*, Vol. 131, pp. 1134–1136 (1974); J. C. Holyrod, J. M. Brodsky, Psychologists' Attitudes and Practices Regarding Erotic and Nonerotic Physical Contact with Patients, *American Psychologist*, Vol. 32, pp. 843–849 (1977).

6. For example, a book has been written about the *Roy v. Hartogs* case. The book, *Betrayal* (Samisdat, 1980) by Clifton Merrit, was later developed into a television docudrama.

7. Stone, The Legal and Ethical Implications of Sexual Activity Between Psychiatrist and Patient, *American Journal of Psychiatry*, Vol. 133, pp. 1138–1141 (1976).

8. Masters and Johnson, Principles of the New Sex Therapy, *American Journal of Psychiatry*, Vol. 133, pp. 548–554 (1976).

9. Dickes and Fleming, *op. cit.*, note 3, p. 328.

10. Representative James Rutkowsky introduced a bill in the Wisconsin legislature that would provide a prison term of up to five years and a $10,000 fine for "therapists— such as psychologists and psychiatrists—who have sexual intercourse with a patient, even with the patient's consent." *Milwaukee Sentinel*, June 7, 1983.

11. Cited in J. Goldstein, A. Dershowitz, and R. D. Schwartz, *Criminal Law: Theory and Process* (Free Press, 1974), pp. 3–23.

12. *People v. Bernstein*, 340 P.2d 299 (1959).

13. Mich. General Laws Annotated Ch. 750.520b(f).

14. *Milwaukee Sentinel, op. cit.*

15. These are unreported jury decisions handed down both in Florida and in California. Personal communication, American Psychiatric Association Committee on Mal-practice.

16. 366 N.Y.S. 297, 300–301 (1975).

17. 263 S.2d 256 (1972).

18. *See, e.g.*, Minn. General Laws Ch. 541.05 (criminal conversation). See also *Felsenthal v. McMillan*, 493 S.W.2d 729 (upholding refusal to grant summary judgment as to cause of action for criminal conversation).

19. Prosser, *Law of Torts*, 4th ed., §124, p. 875.

20. 366 N.Y.S. 297.

21. *Ibid.*

22. *Ibid.*

23. *Zipkin v. Freeman*, 436 S.W.2d 753 (1968).

24. *Hartogs v. Employers Mutual Liability Insurance Company of Wisconsin*, 391 N.Y.S.2d 962 (1977).

25. Dissent in *Roy v. Hartogs*, 366 N.Y.S. 297 (1975).

26. *Ibid.*

27. 366 N.Y.S. 297.

28. *Ibid.*

29. There have been a number of reported appeals from license revocations grounded in sexual impropriety by physicians. Several of these appeals were made by psychia-trists.

30. 15 A.L.R.3d 1173 (1965).

31. American Psychiatric Association, *The Principles of Medical Ethics with Annotations Especially Applicable to Psychiatry*, Washington, D.C., 1981.

32. *Ibid.*

33. *See, e.g.*, Norton, Ethics in Medicine and Law—Standards and Conflicts, *Medical Trial Technique Quarterly*, Spring 1980, p. 377.

34. American Psychiatric Association, *op. cit.* note 31.

35. *See Ceasar v. Mountanos*, 542 F.2d 1064 (9th Cir. 1976).

36. *See* Appelbaum, Confidentiality in Psychiatric Treatment, in L. Grinspoon, ed., *Psychiatry 1982: The American Psychiatric Association Annual Review*, (American Psychiatric Association, 1982).

37. American Psychoanalytic Association, *Principles of Ethics for Psychoanalysts and Provisions for Implementation of the Principles of Ethics for Psychoanalysts*, 1975.

38. *See, e.g.*, Hilberman, *The Rape Victim* (Basic Books, 1976).

39. *See* A. Stanton and M. Schwartz, *The Mental Hospital* (Basic Books, 1954).

40. American Psychoanalytic Association, *op. cit.* note 37.

41. American Psychiatric Association, *op. cit.* note 31.

IX

Psychiatry and Morality:
Three Criticisms

I T IS DIFFICULT, as Erik Erikson has suggested,[1] not to approach the subject of psychiatry and morality with a chip on each shoulder. The very conjunction of the terms is calculated to make blood boil. There are psychiatrists on the one hand who insist that psychiatry is a medical science having nothing to do with morality. And there are philosophers and theologians who are repelled by the thought that modern psychiatry, particularly as influenced by Freud, has anything good or worthwhile to contribute to the subject of morality. I am reminded of a distinguished Harvard philosophy professor who, while attending a symposium on psychoanalysis and philosophy, was so outraged at the very conjunction of these two disciplines he allegedly exclaimed, "Psychoanalysis is a dirty dishpan in the great ocean of philosophy." I have no doubt that if consulted he would express a similar opinion about the conjunction of psychiatry and morality. One can assume that his sentiments would run as follows: the question of morality is the noblest question of mankind involving the possibility of freedom, the grounding of morality in reason, or some ideal of an ordered society. Psychoanalysis and psychiatry, in contrast, are ignoble, small minded, reductionistic, backward looking, even somewhat prurient, and (here I quote the Catholic theologian, Hans Küng) psychoanalysis has "been identified in public opinion with irreligiousness and sexuality, with the breakdown of religion, order, and morality."[2] Many other critics have suggested that modern psychiatry as influenced by Freud is to be blamed for all of the "decadence" of the "permissive society."

These are not just the prejudiced opinions of outsiders. The same views have been echoed by voices within psychoanalysis. Erik Erikson, for example, in his psychohistory *Young Man Luther* writes,

> Neurotic patients and panicky people in general are so starved for beliefs that they will fanatically spread among the unbelievers what are often as yet quite shaky convictions. Because we did not include this fact in our awareness, we were shocked at being called pansexualists. We were distressed at the spread of a compulsive attitude of mutual mental denuding. We were dismayed at a wide-spread fatalism according to which man is nothing but a multiplica-tion of his parents' faults. We must grudgingly admit that even as we were trying to devise, with scientific determinism, a therapy for the few, we were led to promote an ethical disease among the many.[3]

Although there are aspects of this indictment which I think are true and which I shall rely on in my subsequent discussion, I would like to sound a cautionary note. It seems to me that it is too easy to blame too much on Freud. The American hunger for Freud is an appetite which it-self needs to be explained. And there has been a similar loss of moral con-sensus, a similar cynicism about traditional moral authority, and a similar phase of breakdown in conventional religion, order, and morality in societies where Freud and modern psychiatry have had little perceptible influence. But whether or not Erikson is entirely correct about the etiology of the ethical disease, he is certainly ingenuous in asserting that the goal of psychoanalysis was to devise a therapy for the few. That has certainly not been his goal for most of his life, nor was it what inspired Freud's work, from *The Interpretation of Dreams*[4] to *Civilization and Its Discontents*.[5] As Hans Küng rightly observes in *Freud and the Problem of God*, "Psychoanalysis was now applied to literature and aesthetics, to mythology, folklore and educational theory, to prehistory and the history of religion. It was no longer merely a therapeutic procedure but an instrument of universal enlightenment."[6]

I would prefer to describe psychoanalysis as a descriptive develop-mental theory of human subjectivity, but "instrument of enlighten-ment" comes closer to the mark than Erikson's scientific therapy for the few. Modern psychiatry, though less enthusiastic about psychoanalysis than an earlier generation, has been no less ambitious in its general claims to offer universal enlightenment. Particularly, this has been the case in psychiatry's contribution to contemporary problems of morality.

It is difficult to think of a pressing moral question on which psychiatry has not made "authoritative pronouncements." Abortion, capital punishment, racism, sexism, nuclear disarmament, gun control, apartheid, pornography, terrorism, the Vietnam war, euthanasia, poverty, love and marriage—these are only some of the subjects on which we have felt that our professional expertise qualified us to speak. In fact, I should admit to you that I myself have contributed to psychiatric pronouncements on all of these issues. This essay is therefore in some sense confessional—an examination of my own professional conscience. How did psychiatrists presume so much and how is it that we were permitted so much? One President of the American Psychiatric Association using the jargon associated with the Community Mental Health Movement announced to his colleagues that "the world is our catchment area."[7] And he might have added, "Man in the world is our subject matter." He received a standing ovation and went on to become President of the World Psychiatric Association. The grandiosity of modern psychiatry may today seem unjustified, but I believe it can be understood from a certain point of view.

MADNESS, HUMAN NATURE, AND MORALITY

There is in Western thought a long tradition of understanding the human condition in terms of its abnormal manifestations. This tradition is by no means confined to psychiatry. It can be found in such unlikely places as the writings of Immanuel Kant; see for example Kant's *Anthropology from a Pragmatic Point of View*.[8] (I shall be making some comparative comments about Freud and Kant throughout these next two chapters.) The intellectual tradition which Kant exemplifies attempts to isolate the abnormal, madness, at an extreme of the human spectrum as "the most profound degradation of humanity which seems to originate from nature."[9] But having put madness to one side and isolated it, as though it had nothing to do with his understanding of the "normal," Kant's analysis of the situation of the rest of humanity is somehow haunted by the analogy to madness: "To be subject to emotions and passions is probably always an illness of mind because both emotions and passions exclude the sovereignty of reason."[10] For Kant, emotion is akin to "apoplexy" and "passion is delusion." Although Kant had important philosophical justifications for deriving morality from reason, his attempt to do this was set against this conception of passion as delusion. He also, in a way, anticipated contemporary psychiatry's obsession with the problem of self-deception: that we are unaware of our own motives. He wrote, "the veil with which self-love conceals our moral infirmity must be torn away."

Kant, I am sure, believed that the tearing away would be done by a rational moral philosophy, but psychiatry's attribution of self-deception to the unconscious suggested that the veil must be lifted in some other manner. One of psychiatry's most convincing claims that it has a right to participate in moral discourse is bottomed on this assertion of unconscious self-deception. For example, many psychiatrists believe we have a professional as well as personal justification for becoming involved in the movement for nuclear disarmament. We argue that many people are denying, repressing, or supressing the frightening possibility of an atomic holocaust. These psychological mechanisms, which in this instance lead to moral and political inertia, are, we assert, a classic example of pathological self-deception. I shall return to this theme. But here let me just emphasize that to claim that someone is practicing self-deception, if it is to be a powerful claim, must also mean that the psychiatrist sees through the self-deception to the truth of the matter, what in fact lies concealed behind the veil of self-deception. To know that is to know something about the "meaning of life."

At any rate, it should be clear that the attempt to understand human nature in the metaphors of madness and self-deception did not begin with modern psychiatry. Freud would use language identical to Kant's: "The id is the place of passions" and the ego, of "reason and sanity."[11] The tradition to which Kant and Freud belong sees the peril of humanity in the triumph of passion over judgment and reason. This tradition accepts the basic dichotomy of reason and passion as a given in human nature. Passion at war with reason remains even today one of the most compelling paradigms both of mental abnormality and of the human condition.

Modern biological psychiatry grounded in twentieth century medical science has little professed interest in this rational humanist tradition. However, its practitioners share Kant's opinion that madness originates from nature, and they agree with Kant's view that "the germ of derangement develops together with the germ of reproduction and is thus hereditary."[12] But if madness is biological and genetic, how shall we understand the rest of the disorders of consciousness that stretch from madness on one side to normal human suffering on the other?

Some psychiatrists have argued that this question is no longer our business: the old psychiatry, they say, is dead; madness is part of the neurosciences; the rest is the human condition.[13] But even as biological psychiatrists say this, they are busily engaged in studying the whole spectrum of the disorders of consciousness and charting the biological substrate of the human condition. Nor are they hesitant to extend the reach of biologically determined mental illness further and further from the extreme of madness. And if we look to practice rather than theory, we find everywhere the prescription of chemicals to ease the pain and suffering of the human condition. Through the prism of medical science, the passions of everyday life become symptoms to be treated chemically. In analogy to Kant, biological psychiatry, after declaring madness a biological disorder, is haunted by biology in its understanding of the rest of humanity. The problem is and has always been for psychiatry—is it only a theory of madness or is it also a more general theory of human nature? Or is it even possible in principle to make such a distinction? Can one explain madness without explaining human nature?

What is important is that when psychiatry begins to gain popular acceptance as in fact providing a theory of human nature, it begins to establish the context of moral action and moral obligation. It does this in at least two obvious ways. First, most Western notions of morality require as a fundamental premise the existence of a unified and continuous self and a will. Philosophers who construct theories of morality recognize the need to ground these fundamental premises on some assumptions about mind and mental functioning—a psychology, no matter how limited, is required. One can demonstrate this need for a psychology not only in Kant, but in such contrasting moralists as St. Augustine in his *Confessions*[14] and Sartre in *Being and Nothingness*.[15] If morality must be constructed on a psychology, as I believe, then profound changes in the accepted psychology inescapably raise questions about the accepted morality. Modern psychiatry as influenced by Freud seems to many observers to have produced just that result. Sartre recognized this and went to great lengths to repudiate the central Freudian construct of unconscious self-deception and to replace it with the formidable moral notion of bad faith.[16]

A second way in which modern psychiatry established the context of moral action and obligation was by producing convincing stories about what it means to be a person. It did this by "uncovering" the "true history" of human drives and by revealing in Ricoeur's phrase "the archaeology of desire."[17]

Psychoanalysis not only challenged the unity of the self, it privileged a certain account of virtues and vices which made the will a minor actor in the moral drama of life. Though there was for academics much to criticize in these Freudian revelations, they had a compelling influ-ence on popular psychology and mass culture. Freudianism could not be kept out of the dialogue on the "Meaning of Life."

From the moment American psychiatry embraced Freud, it had a unified theory of human nature, from which its explanations of mental disorder and treatment could be derived. That, I believe, is what Freud intended, contrary to what Erikson suggests. If modern psychiatry started down the path that Kant and other theorists of human nature had taken, guided by Freud, we reached a different destination. Modern psychiatry produced a vision of human nature in which morality was itself a passion at war with reason. Moral choices and decisions were based on unconscious determinants, all of which seemed incompatible with Kant's idea of free moral agents choosing between right and wrong. Erikson wants to write this off as a kind of misunderstanding, a premature acceptance of tentative conclusions. But Freud intended on the basis of his theory of human nature to throw down the gauntlet at the idea of man as a free moral agent. What else could Freud have meant when he embraced Groddeck's words, "We are lived by unknown and uncontrollable forces,"[18] or when he placed Kant's categorical impera-tive in the id as the legacy of a phylogenetic past? The morality which had power over men came not from any higher authority, not from reason, but from an unknown moral passion, a stranger within. Immoral-ity was equally mysterious and required deciphering.

THREE PERSPECTIVES ON PSYCHIATRY AND MORALITY

Generations of American psychiatrists have tried to find ways around what more and more of them came to recognize as problematic and embarrassing. The most well-known and beloved American popularizer of Freud's ideas, Karl Menninger, was moved to wonder, *Whatever Became of Sin?*[19] But it is not just psychoanalysis in modern psychiatry that called into question the ideal of a free moral agent. All of the dominant conceptual paradigms of modern psychiatry—biological, be-havioral, psychodynamic, and social—conflict with traditional ideas about free moral agents. Although I am sure philosophers would say this bald statement of conflict is wrong, I am equally sure they would disagree on just how it is wrong. At least for psychiatrists who explain behavior in terms of biological transmethylation, reinforcement sched-ules, defective superegos, and demographic trends, there is still no convincing resolution of this problem.

Perhaps the most obvious practical implication of explaining morality and immorality in terms of the unconscious, the reinforcement schedule, or the DNA and undermining the ideal conception of free moral agents choosing to do right or wrong is that it undermines the theory of our criminal law. It makes it much more difficult to attribute moral blameworthiness to those who break the law or who in some way offend.

As Lord Devlin stated it, "Everywhere the concept of sickness expands at the expense of the concept of moral responsibility."[20] The concept of moral responsibility, of course, is what justifies punishment. Viewed from this perspective, modern psychiatry appeared as the antagonist of the principle of retributive punishment. It joined forces with Christian forgiveness in a secular version of "to understand is to forgive." Christopher Lasch makes Lord Devlin's point with more sweeping rhetoric: "But it is precisely this universal understanding, sympathy, and tolerance (which in any case does not conceal the persistence of intolerance at a deeper level) that reflect the collapse of moral consensus, the collapse of distinctions between right and wrong, the collapse of moral authority. . . . "[21] But if psychiatry as influenced by Freud made people uncomfortable about punishing sinners, it soon became clear that in the alternative to punishment more was involved than simple forgiveness.

Reviewing Karl Menninger's book, *The Crime of Punishment*,[22] the late Professor Packer of Stanford Law School suggested that the impulse to treat and the impulse to punish originated in the same region of the psyche. Foucault argues that at the end of the Middle Ages evil went out of the world and madness came in.[23] One might, in that vein, say about twentieth century America that progressivism and psychiatry drove retribution out of our moral deliberations and replaced it with treatment. Many critics began to find similar evidence that psychiatry, far from being a threat to conventional social morality, had become the very instrument of that morality. The criticism came from an entirely different direction than Erikson anticipated. Indeed, Erikson was himself a target of this attack. Far from being a corrupter of conventional social morality (or a liberating influence), psychoanalysis and psychiatry were identified as the chief vehicles of conventional social morality of oppression and of passing judgment on people. Of course this can be partly explained away in historical terms: the vanguard of social change had passed Freud by. The Freudian revolution becomes, over time, a counterrevolution; what was liberating for one generation becomes oppressive for the next. Another way to think of this is that Freud's descriptive theory of human nature was seized on, particularly in the

United States, as a prescriptive theory. This is one way to account for the grandiosity of modern psychiatry: all deviance became a disease, including crime and immorality, and the psychiatrist presides over the diagnosis and the cure. At any rate, we now have encountered three perspectives on the involvement of psychiatry in moral issues. First, there is the notion that psychiatry, particularly as influenced by Freud, undermined the consensus of conventional social morality and traditional moral authority. Second, that psychiatry embodied and enforced conventional social morality and authority. Finally, that psychiatry undercuts our fundamental conception of free moral agents whom we can justly punish. I shall attempt to offer a partial account of how all this happens.

Thomas Szasz, a psychiatrist and psychoanalyst himself, who is the author of *The Myth of Mental Illness*,[24] *The Manufacture of Madness*,[25] and *Law, Liberty, and Psychiatry*,[26] has made all three of these arguments against psychiatry.

(1) In *The Myth of Mental Illness*, he argues that Freud transformed what was in essence a kind of cheating, malingering and lying into an illness, hysteria.

(2) In *The Manufacture of Madness*, he describes psychiatry as the continuation of the inquisition—"the defense of the dominant ethic." Just as the inquisition invented witches, psychiatry invented the holy myth of schizophrenia.

(3) Throughout his writing he repeatedly attacks every psychiatric paradigm that undercuts the traditional view of the free moral agent. He is particularly obdurate in his demand that the insanity defense be abolished. Even the most obviously deranged person intends the consequences of his acts and to deny this is to deny that person's humanity. Although Szasz sometimes makes this claim as though it were an empirical fact, at other times it seems to be a normative or ideal view of human nature. In order to maintain this view, Szasz has declared that even Kant is wrong about the extreme of madness. There is no mental illness, everything is the human condition. Perhaps the essence of Szasz's criticism is that psychiatry is nothing but ideology masquerading as scientific objectivity.

FREUD'S INFLUENCE

Although Foucault suggests in *Madness and Civilization* that these charges against psychiatry have been true since the Middle Ages, the psychiatrist was at the periphery of society until the twentieth century. It was Freud who turned the attention of psychiatry from the mad-houses to the middle class. It is against Freud and his influence that the ideological arguments are made. Although Freud had very little experi-ence with psychotics himself, in the course of his work he conceived a coherent unified psychological theory of mental illness. He broke through the dividing line between the most profound degradation of humanity at one end and between the normal and the neurotic at the other end. One can no longer think of a continuum from madness to sanity; normality is no longer on the continuum. Freud literally believed that neurosis was the price we pay for civilization. Although American Freudians sacrificed this idea on the altar of therapeutic optimism, Freud had declared normality a nearly unattainable ideal. In this respect, I doubt that he differed very much from Kant or from certain other moral philosophers, if you allow me to analogize between Kant's assessment of the moral infirmity of mankind due to the veil of self-love and Freud's assessment of our neurotic infirmity due to the veil of unconscious repression.

There is another distinction in Freud's thought which is essential to my analysis. Freud believed that there were no qualitative differences between the mental processes of the psychotic and the rest of us. Ultimately, the only distinctions were quantitative. The only difference between a delusion and a fantasy was quantity. The only difference between a memory and a hallucination was quantity. Psychosis was dreaming while awake. Everyone had all variations of the Oedipus complex. The difference between heterosexual and homosexual was quantitative. I think it was Goethe who said that no man ever had a fan-tasy that I have not had. Freud would have said that the claim was believable.

But there is something deeply problematic with a theory which, though it provides us an understanding of all mental processes, normal and abnormal, relies on unspecified quantities to explain all of the differences. This problem of quantity becomes more troubling when we recognize that the determinist conception of Freudian theory is grounded on these mysterious quantities which impel fantasy, emotion, thought, and behavior. In the end it is not clear whether Freud placed the categorical imperative in the id and rejected the notion of free moral agents based on empirical observations of how people actually behave—that is, some empirical view of human nature—or on some *a priori* assumption about human nature derived from the determinist theory of science. He often seems to be saying both at once. This, you will recognize, is the criticism I made of Szasz, only from the other direction. I believe that in both instances these are simply different intuitions about what it means to be a person. The way Freud imposed this intuition on his theory is by invoking the quantitative factor. In fact, the quantitative factor can be used as a red flag as one reads Freud, marking the places where descriptions of mental processes and subjective experiences are transformed into explanatory determinist theories. The quantitative factor is central to the hydraulic theory of emotions, to the catharsis theory of therapy, and to Freud's mean conception of the human possibilities of freedom and love. It is on the basis of the quantitative factor that Freud ridiculed the biblical injunction to love thy neighbor, and the more mysterious injunction to love thine enemy.[27]

If one deprives Freud of this quantitative factor, one can no longer claim for him that he offers either a coherent theoretical explanation of mental disorder or a compelling account of human nature. The strongest claim one can make is that it is a description of a kind of subjective experience, the history of desire in the individual rendered in a determinist and selfless discourse.

Freud said that neurotics suffer from reminiscences, and we might say that reminiscences were Freud's subject matter. *Not* man in the world, but man and his reminiscences. Out of that subject matter one cannot get a complete explanation of the human condition or perhaps even a correct understanding of one of Freud's most important subjects, *guilt*.

But having said all these things (and there are other critical things to say about Freud), I find it hard to reject his most basic contribution to Western thought, the dynamic unconscious. After Richard Nixon had lost the presidential election to John F. Kennedy, he came back to California and eventually ran for Governor of the State. Everywhere Nixon went on his campaign trail, reporters would ask the obvious question, was he running for Governor in order to run again for President? Finally, after having been asked this again and again, Nixon at one press conference drew himself up, looked the reporter in the eye, and said, "Listen, I would like to tell the press once and for all to please stop asking this question; I can assure you that I will be fully satisfied if I am elected Governor of the United States." We all now understand this error in a Freudian perspective, namely that the conscious and the mental are not identical, and I think most of us have some feeling that we do not fully understand ourselves and that we are all capable of similar revealing Freudian errors. The basis of the psychoanalyst's claim to special knowledge is that by his methods he has access to our unconscious and understands the processes by which our repressed desires become known. We are trapped in our self-deceptions, and the psychoanalyst can see through us to the truth of the matter. We must now examine this supposed truth because in it are the concealed human values and the moral postures which have had such a great influence on modern life. It is by contributing the dynamic unconscious to our understanding of what it means to be a person that psychoanalysis has had its greatest influence on morality.

Freud believed that the truth about the unconscious and the shaping of personality, conscience, and passion came from two major sources—infantile experiences which were repressed to comprise infantile amnesia and the phylogenetic unconscious, including the core of the superego. This phylogenetic element was Freud's sociobiology, and in retrospect it seems entirely speculative. Modern Freudians have tried to read this sociobiology out of Freud, but it was a crucial aspect of his theory and it was pervasive. It could not be removed by clean theoretical surgery, and it contained the hidden ideology of psychoanalysis. It is equally important to recognize that Freud's theory of infantile experiences was only dubiously empirical; it was also structured by sociobiological assumptions and by Freud's intuitions about what it means to be a person.

It was Freud's sociobiological assumptions and his emphasis on early infantile experiences within the family that allowed him to construct a theory of what it meant to be a person which was transcultural and transhistorical.[28] The limitations of such a theory and the errors in Freud's sociobiology now seem obvious to us. We recognize that what Freud understood to be the truth of the matter is to a large extent ideological, and nowhere is this more obvious than in Freud's truth about women.

Before turning to that, let me summarize and reformulate my thoughts. I have been trying to think through with you some of the moral ramifications of modern psychiatry; at the same time I have a more basic question—is it possible to have a theory of mental illness which does not imply a theory of human nature and which in turn contextualizes the problem of morality? Now, it is possible to minimize the apparent moral implications of psychiatry by limiting mental illness to an extreme, as Kant and some contemporary biological psychiatrists would do. Madness comes from nature, and the rest of our disorders, perhaps, from living. But even those who draw such lines find it difficult to keep the domains of madness and the human condition separate. By examining Freud, I hoped to show the most powerful example of psychiatry's attempt to give a coherent unified theory of mental disorder and human nature and to tell us what it means to be a person. If one accepts and applies these theories as valid self-descriptions, one also accepts the values and moral postures concealed in them. The appeal of Freud's theories to twentieth century men and women as revealing self descriptions is ultimately the key to Freud's influence on contemporary morality. Even Jean Paul Sartre, who made elaborate arguments against Freud's unconscious and who created his own existential psychoanalysis partly in reaction to Freud, when it came to writing his own autobiography, took as a central theme a Freudian self-description. Sartre reports that a psychoanalyst had told him that because his father had died when Sartre was an infant, Sartre did not have a superego. This seems to have delighted Sartre. He wrote that other men went through life weighted down by their fathers "like Aeneas carrying Anchises from the walls of Troy," but he, the philosopher of radical freedom, had no such burden.[29]

If Freud's theories were attractive as valid self-descriptions even for philosophers skeptical of Freud, they were enormously attractive to bourgeois American men and women. Or as Kate Millett, the radical feminist, suggests, they were the ideas with which American men and women were indoctrinated. She writes, "The new formulation of old attitudes (bourgeois, patriarchical moralism) had to come from science, and particularly from the emerging social sciences . . . [These replaced religion and traditional morality and were] the most useful and authoritative branches of social control and manipulation . . . New prophets arrived on the scene. The most influential of these was Sigmund Freud, beyond question the strongest individual counterrevolutionary force in the ideology of sexual politics."[30]

Freud summarized most of his theories about women in a brief lecture on "Femininity." He begins by demonstrating that it is impossible to define male and female; therefore, "Psychoanalysis does not try to describe what a woman is—that would be a task it could scarcely perform—but sets about inquiring how she comes into being, how a woman develops out of a child with bisexual disposition."[31] But Freud does not in fact begin his description of the course of a woman's development with a bisexual child. As his many critics have repeatedly pointed out, Freud's little girl is a bisexual defective boy. The supposed travails of this defective boy in reaching adult feminine sexuality are well known. The ultimate achievement of mature female sexuality was a rare event in Freud's view. There were other consequences of Freud's theory of how woman "comes into being": her weak superego, her failures of sublimation, her envy, and her deficiencies in a sense of justice. The woman who did internalize these Freudian self-descriptions would assuredly think of herself as erotically and morally inferior to men. But despite the many criticisms of these theories, many women did internalize them as valid self-descriptions, particularly Freud's ideal of mature female sexuality. This Freudian truth about female sexuality, based on a speculative sociobiology, was widely accepted as a correct self-description. It led millions of women to believe that they were sexually inadequate, a conclusion that millions of their husbands shared. For decades women would be told that their sexual "problem" was a manifestation of their masculine protest, as was their wish to have a career.

As a psychiatrist and psychoanalyst who has lived through all of the things I have been describing, you can perhaps imagine how discomforting all this has been. Freud's theory of human nature had been shown to be unnatural. Ironically, we were wrong about sexuality. The subject is more complicated, and the answers are still more elusive than Freud imagined. And if we were wrong about that, what else was wrong? When we penetrated the patient's veil of self-love and self-deception, what we had found was not the truth of the matter, but our own ideology. And we had been guilty of a certain kind of immorality ourselves. We had treated our patients' own self-descriptions as false. Indeed, the basic therapeutic posture of the psychiatrist raised moral questions because it was grounded on the premise that we should treat much of what the patient said about himself as self-deception.[32]

I shall have more to say about the moral aspects of the therapeutic relationship itself: the problems of domination, the undercurrents of love, and the risks of vulnerability and attachment. But for now it should be clear that the supposedly nonjudgmental psychoanalyst had as the framework of his understanding of illness and treatment a prescriptive theory. That prescriptive theory was in many respects an ideology which some critics argued was designed or applied for the purpose of rationalizing interpersonal oppression of women by men, homosexuals by heterosexuals, and rebels by conservatives.

CAN IDEOLOGY BE AVOIDED?

These criticisms raised questions not only about the enterprise of therapy, but also about the whole conception of mental illness in American psychiatry. As attempts were made to revise the psychodynamic conception of mental illness by removing what was considered offensive, the explanatory power of Freud's theory of mental illness was lost. Psychiatry has entered a period in which there are no convincing connections between the diagnoses described in our Diagnostic Manual and our explanations of those diagnoses.[33] Increasingly, we agree that the extreme of madness has a biological explanation, but as to the rest of the disorders of consciousness there is a struggle of competing views. Simple depression, for example, might be the result of an enzyme disturbance, a cognitive disorder of self-image, an unconscious introject, or a consequence of social isolation and alienation. The treatment the patient received depended to a large extent on the psychiatrist's commitment to one of these approaches. Some psychiatrists seem to think there are four kinds of simple depression depending on which of these etiological elements dominate. Others are eclectic, and the patient will be met at the door by a team of clinicians each applying a different approach. Each of these four paradigms—biological, behavioral, psycho-dynamic, and social—has its own problematic moral implications. But when they are all put together, there is no coherent vision of the human condition and there is considerable confusion about what kinds of moral judgments are being made or evaded. If this is true for all of these paradigms put together, it is also particularly true for the psychodynamic paradigm.

Without a unifying theory about the truth behind self-deception, more and more psychodynamic psychiatrists are attracted to the possibil-ity of listening to their patients without any theoretical preconceptions. Even if this is possible, and even if the therapist avoids imposing his definition of what it means to be a person on the patient, there are still inescapable moral implications to this enterprise.

Many of our patients seek help in situations where they are struggling not just with depression, stress, or anxiety but also with moral problems. Should they get a divorce? Should they fight for custody of their children? Should they leave a job where they are needed and should they have made a commitment for one that pays more? Should they tell their spouse about their affair? Should they put their parents in a nursing home?

Psychiatrists tend to think that if we allow our patients to ventilate their feelings it will help them not only to understand themselves but also to attain greater clarity in making these moral decisions. The psychiatrist, without expressing his own potentially oppressive moral convictions or ideology, will help the patient get in touch with what seems right for him. But what seems right is often a conclusion reached as the result of exploring repressed desires and weighing competing inclinations. It is a kind of reflection in which the outside world shrinks and the self expands. This may be the correct way to get in touch with unconscious desires and to identify self-destructive impulses, but is it a sensible way to frame moral questions for oneself? Can moral questions be framed and resolved in a process where the self looms large and the world seems small?

I remember a patient, the wife of a scientist, who had several children. Her husband, she felt, was remote even on the rare instances when he was home. The patient came to me troubled about her unsatisfactory marriage. I encouraged her to explore her feelings and did little more than listen compassionately for two hours a week. Within six weeks, this woman had met a wonderful new man, a real companion, was happily in love, and had decided to leave her husband and four children. Now regardless of whether this was good or bad, right or wrong, it seemed that I and the process of therapy were partly responsible both for her newly found great happiness and her moral decisions, all of which she ceremonialized by unexpectedly bringing her new friend to the therapy hour for my seal of approval. Human problems do not come packaged in psychiatric bits and moral bits. It seems that there may be a moral cost even in nonjudgmental listening. Clearly, cultural bias and concealed moral assumptions played a part in the fallacies of the theory of psychoanalysis. But is it possible that the introspective method of free association is itself a major factor in painting the false picture of human nature? After all, it is on reminiscences—free association—and not man in the world that the theoretical edifice was built.

FREUD, KANT, AND FREE ASSOCIATION

Freud asked his patient to give free rein to his thoughts and report "everything that comes into his head, even if it is *disagreeable* for him to say it, even if it seems to him *unimportant* or actually *nonsensical*." If the patient allows himself to free-associate, "he will present us with a mass of material—subject to the influence of the unconscious." That influence can then be examined and deciphered so that the patient comes to understand himself.[34]

But more than a century before Freud discovered this fundamental rule of psychoanalysis, Kant had considered and rejected it. He writes in the *Anthropology*,

> To scrutinize the various acts of the imagination within me, when I call them forth, is indeed worth reflection, as well as necessary and useful for logic and metaphysics. But to wish to play the spy upon one's self, when those acts come to mind unsummoned and of their own accord (which happens through the play of the unpremedita-tively creative imagination) is to reverse the natural order of the cognitive powers since then the rational elements do not take the lead (as they should) but instead follow behind. This desire for self investigation is either already a disease of the mind (hypochondria) or will lead to such a disease and ultimately to the madhouse. . . . He who has a great deal to tell of inner experiences (for example of grace temptations etc.) may, in the course of his voyage to self-discovery, have made his first landing only at Anticyra [the land of the insane].[35]

Although I do not entirely share Kant's opinion about "the natural order of the cognitive powers" or about the negative value of such "self discovery," it may be that he is right as far as its value for framing moral questions. There is a tradition in moral philosophy of stepping back after you have attempted to explore and understand the facts of the situation, and then attempting to reexamine the case at hand in terms of some broader moral principle. But psychiatry has no such tradition of stepping back and no generally accepted moral principles if it did. Kant made these observations about free association in the *Anthropology*, where he argued that psychology generally would get nowhere so long as it relied on introspection. He advised psychologists to develop an anthropological method based on systematic observations of men and women in the world. He then offers the fruit of some of his own systematic observations. Although one can find evidence of Kant's uncontestable genius in this book, it is clear to any modern reader that Kant, this preeminent figure in Western moral philosophy, had nothing in his store of rational morality to protect his systematic observations against his own personal biases and cultural prejudices, some of which he shared with Freud (particularly his attitudes toward women). The philosopher who introduces the English translation of Kant's *Anthropology* is "amazed at [Kant's] uncritical views" and asserts that "any failure on [Kant's] part to live up to the moral ideal must be ascribed to a lack of experience which permitted his prejudices to remain unde-tected."[36] But one might ask, what then would correct Kant's "lack of experience"?

STEPPING BACK AND GUILT

Freud subjectively explored the unconscious and found his own biases. Kant objectively observed his fellow man and found his own biases. Is there no solution to this problem? If there is, I have not yet found it. But I do have a sense of what has been missing from my own moral vision as a psychiatrist and psychoanalyst. First, I think we must recognize that even the most neutral and compassionate psychotherapy potentially misframes moral questions. We have to begin by acknowledging that to ourselves and to our patients. (Psychoanalysts in days gone by used to insist that their patients make no major life decisions during the process of psychoanalysis. The pace of life has quickened, and it is difficult to maintain this requirement.) Next, we have to think of ways of stepping back, or better helping our patients to step back, so that moral questions can come into focus. Second, we must rethink our conception of guilt. If the psychotherapeutic situation does not bring moral problems into focus for the patient, it may also be true that the psychotherapeutic situation prejudices the attempt to set out the context of morality.

I want to argue that there is a crucial confusion in modern psychiatry which has arisen in this way which has to do with our understanding of depression, guilt, and what Freud called moral anxiety. What we see in our depressed patients (and who is not "depressed"?) has little or nothing to do with moral obligations to others. This "superego" is not the inner voice of morality or the categorical imperative: it is the voice of self-loathing. The same patient who is tortured by what Freud called moral anxiety as he reflects on his life has little or no sense of his moral obligations to anyone else; in fact his self-loathing typically stands in the way of his moral ambitions and obligations. The patient will say that he is tortured by compulsive ideas, that he is really a fraud and worthless even though he is a distinguished professor at a great university. His psychoanalyst will say about this man that he has a strict superego which has initiated a critical moral attack upon his ego. But this professor typically has the same view of everyone else. If he has a strict superego, it is not an inner voice commanding moral obligations, duty, or kindness to others. This voice from the unconscious is not the voice of morality, it is the voice of self-loathing. Psychiatry influenced by Freud has confused self-loathing and moral conscience.

I once complained to a distinguished philosopher that he had failed to honor an obligation he had made to me. His immediate response was, "I thought you psychiatrists are supposed to help people *not* to feel guilty." He said this with a smile, but I think his humorous sally bespeaks the real confusion in ordinary language. Psychiatry needs to rethink the subject of guilt, and we need to begin with a careful distinction between self-loathing—arising because the self is not as perfect, as powerful, and as lovable as the person believes it should be— and guilt, which arises because one has failed in one's moral obligations to others. Of course, the enterprise of conceptualizing what it means to have moral obligations is not one that psychiatry can embark upon alone. But hopefully, in the future, psychiatry will be one of a family of disciplines which knows that to study human nature is to study moral obligations. This enterprise will help us to remember what Kant learned from Rousseau: "What is truly permanent in human nature is not any condition in which it once existed and from which it has fallen, rather it is the goal for which and toward which it moves."[37]

REFERENCES

1. E. Erikson, *Young Man Luther* (Norton, 1958), p. 21.

2. H. Küng, *Freud and the Problem of God* (Yale University Press, 1980), p. 55.

3. Erikson, *op. cit.*, p. 19.

4. S. Freud, *The Interpretation of Dreams* (Basic Books, 1955).

5. S. Freud, *Civilization and Its Discontents*, standard ed. (Hogarth Press, 1961).

6. Küng, *op. cit.*, p. 27.

7. Cited in A. Stone, Response to the Presidential Address, *American Journal of Psychiatry*, Vol. 136, pp. 1020–1022 (1979).

8. I. Kant, *Anthropology from a Pragmatic Point of View* (Southern Illinois University Press, 1978).

9. *Ibid.*, p. 112.

10. *Ibid.*, p. 251.

11. S. Freud, *The Ego and the Id and Other Works*, translated by J. Strachey, standard ed., Vol. 19 (Hogarth Press, 1927).

12. Kant, *op. cit.*, p. 115.

13. E. F. Torrey, *The Death of Psychiatry* (Penguin, 1975).

14. Saint Augustine, *Confessions*, translated by E. B. Pusey (Dent, 1966).

15. J. P. Sartre, *Being and Nothingness: An Essay on Phenomenological Ontology*, translated by H. E. Barnes (Philosophical Library, 1956).

16. See particularly, *Ibid.*, Part I, Chapter 2, "Bad Faith," and Part IV, Chapter 2, "Doing and Having."

17. P. Ricoeur, *Freud and Philosophy: An Essay on Interpretation*, translated by D. Savage (Yale University Press, 1970).

18. Freud, *The Ego and the Id, op. cit.*, p. 23.

19. K. Menninger, *Whatever Became of Sin?* (Hawthorn Books, 1973).

20. P. Devlin, *The Enforcement of Morals* (Oxford University Press, 1959), p. 17.

21. C. Lasch, *Haven in a Heartless World: The Family Besieged* (Basic Books, 1977), p. 221.

22. K. Menninger, *The Crime of Punishment* (Viking Press, 1968).

23. M. Foucault, *Madness and Civilization: A History of Insanity in the Age of Reason*, translated by R. Howard (Pantheon Books, 1965).

24. T. Szasz, *The Myth of Mental Illness: Foundations of a Theory of Personal Conduct*, rev. ed. (Harper and Row, 1974).

25. T. Szasz, *The Manufacture of Madness: A Comparative Study of the Inquisition and the Mental Health Movement* (Harper and Row, 1970).

26. T. Szasz, *Law, Liberty and Psychiatry: An Inquiry into the Social Uses of Mental Health Practices* (Macmillan, 1963).

27. S. Freud, *Civilization and its Discontents, op. cit.*, p. 109.

28. H. Marcuse, *Eros and Civilization: A Philosophical Inquiry into Freud* (Beacon Press, 1955) (see especially Epilogue, "Critique of Neo-Freudian Revisionism").

29. J. P. Sartre, *The Words*, translated by B. Frechtman (G. Brazilier, 1964).

30. K. Millett, *Sexual Politics* (Doubleday, 1970), p. 178.

31. S. Freud, Femininity, *New Introductory Lectures on Psychoanalysis* (1933), translated by J. Strachey (Norton, 1964), p. 116.

32. S. Bok, *Address to American Psychiatric Association*, New Orleans, May 1981.

33. A. Stone, Presidential Address: Conceptual Ambiguity and Morality in Modern Psychiatry, *American Journal of Psychiatry*, Vol. 137, pp. 887–893 (1980).

34. S. Freud, *Outline of Psychoanalysis*, standard ed., Vol. 23 (Hogarth Press, 1964), p. 174.

35. Kant, *op. cit.*, p. 17.

36. *Ibid.*, Introduction, F. P. Van Der Pitte, pp. xix, xx.

37. E. Cassirer, *Rousseau, Kant, Goethe: Two Essays*, translated by J. Gutmann, et al. (Princeton University Press, 1970), p. 20.

X

Psychiatry as Morality

I N THE PREVIOUS CHAPTER I described how modern psychiatry has been criticized: first, for undermining conventional morality, then for enforcing conventional morality, and more generally for under-cutting what seems to be essential to moral theory—the idea of an autonomous person choosing between good and evil. I suggested that the reason these criticisms were tenable was that modern psychiatry presented itself as offering not just a theory of mental disorder, but also a theory of the human condition. This theory of the human condition contained certain moral postures and established a context for moral ambition.

At the same time, I was working through my own critique of psychoanalysis as a dominant theory of the human condition in Ameri-can psychiatry. My analysis of that critique might have been easier to follow if I had begun by considering the method of Freud's "discovery," the situation in which the patient is asked to free-associate. I argued that this method develops a certain kind of evidence which prejudices the attempt to construct a theory of the human condition. I suggested that Freud's theory based on that evidence is not an explanation of the person in the world but rather a developmental description of human subjectivity. Two other ideas were important to this critique. First, that the way Freud made his descriptive theory seem like an explanatory theory was by invoking mysterious quantities. For example, it may be true that when we reminisce and free-associate about our parents we do evoke sensual feelings about them and fearful, hostile memories as well. It may even be true, as I think it is, that everyone who reminisces will eventually come upon such memories. But the mystery of how those memories explain our personality, our lives, and our current behaviors remains a mystery because Freud invoked an unknown quantitative factor as the crucial explanatory element in the connection.

The other point I tried to make is that the psychotherapeutic setting in which the self looms large and the world small is not an appro-priate setting *in which* to frame moral questions or *from which* to conceptualize the possibilities of human morality. Psychiatrists are called head shrinkers, but from this perspective it is the world and not the head they shrink. I suggested two ways for changing this predica-ment, one clinical and one theoretical. At the clinical level, it is necessary to acknowledge the problem and to develop a method for stepping back and reexamining human problems in a moral perspective. At the level of theory, it is necessary to reconceptualize the superego and the idea of guilt. I distinguished between self-loathing arising out of the failure of the self to be perfect, powerful, or lovable and guilt that one has failed in one's moral obligations to others. The former is the theme of narcissism and the latter of moral obligation. At the most general level I wanted to suggest that psychiatry has contributed to the general acceptance of a kind of discourse about the moral adventure of life, in which the veil of self-love has not been torn away. Self-love has instead been reinterpreted as self-fulfillment or self-actualization.

The problem with self-fulfillment and self-actualization, like the problem of narcissism, is that these can be lonely modes of existence. If Freud's neurotics suffered from reminiscences, today our patients suffer from loneliness.

There was another theme that I want to reemphasize. The basic premise of any psychiatry that posits an unconscious is that the patient's own self-description is a self-deception. The power and significance of this premise depends on whether the psychiatrist truly knows what lies behind the self-deception. I gave the example of Freud's truth about women to demonstrate that we did not know the truth about self-deception. Nonetheless, I continue to believe that the dynamic uncon-scious is real, that self-deception is crucial, and that if psychiatry is to understand the human condition it must understand self-deception. The problem is that with this presumption of the patient's self-deception, psychiatry teeters on the threshold of paternalism and of disrespect for the person.

The charge of paternalism today confounds the psychiatrist at every turn. Whether treatment is voluntary or involuntary, whether it is a matter of diagnosis or prescription, whether the treatment helps or not, every interaction between psychiatrist and patient has taken on this political and controversial dimension of paternalism. If you disagreed with Freud for telling his women patients that their striving in the world outside the home was a masculine protest based on penis envy, you may agree with Karen Horney. She, in refuting Freud's influence, told her women patients who wanted to be good mothers and homemak-ers to live lives more like men, because modern women invest too much of themselves in love and thus leave themselves too vulnerable to rejection and loss of self-esteem.[1] But whatever your opinion may be of these two kinds of advice, you will acknowledge that both are implicitly a kind of paternalistic or maternalistic moral instruction implying that the patient has deceived herself about her goals in life, and when the self-deception is stripped away, the psychiatrist knows more about the true goals of women and the ideal relation between the sexes.

If psychiatrists still practice moral instruction in the sense that they help patients to decide how to live their lives, from where do they get their vision of morality? Do they derive it from their psychological understanding of human nature? Do they import into psychiatry their own unexamined moral attitudes and beliefs? Or do they, as some claim, remain neutral and nonjudgmental, working entirely within the context of the patient, applying only the patient's values and moral convictions as they emerge in therapy? Philip Rieff in his book, *Freud: The Mind of the Moralist*,[2] suggests that Freud had a moral perspective which derived from his theory of therapy. What this "penultimate morality" amounts to is the duty to examine the history and the development of one's moral convictions. Rieff's underlying assumption about Freud's morality might be expressed as follows: human beings typically cling to some childlike illusory ideal (the parent as god-like redeemer and moral authority). When they come into analysis, they project that illusory ideal onto the analyst. This parental ideal is somehow tied up with a person's deepest moral convictions, which are typically unexamined. During analysis he will work through his attachment to this ideal, reconsider his moral convictions, face up to reality and necessity, and relinquish his illusions, including the illusion of moral authority as symbolized by the omnipotent father. Life without illusions is the goal of this penultimate morality. And it is an appropriate morality for a man whose work can be understood as a revolutionary criticism of the world he knew. It is Freud's relentless pursuit of this vision which has led critics to say that Freud's inspiration lacked all of the religious virtues: faith, hope, and charity.

THE MORAL PREMISES OF PSYCHOTHERAPISTS

But if Freud offered only self-knowledge, there have been other psychotherapists willing to go beyond the analysis of illusions. They offer explicit moral instruction based on their psychological theories. Let me give you a published example. This happens to be from a well-known psychologist. His patient has reported her guilt about not doing enough for her parents. Her father had a long history of alcoholism, her mother had had breast cancer surgery, and there had been other long drawn-out family problems. The patient feels she has no life of her own. The patient reportedly says, "I was brought up with that! You always have to give of yourself. If you think of yourself, you're wrong." To this the therapist responds, "Now, why do you have to keep believing that—at your age? You believed a lot of superstitions when you were younger. Why do you have to retain them? We can see why your parents would have to indoctrinate you with this kind of nonsense, because that's their belief. But why do you still have to believe this nonsense—that one should be devoted to others, self-sacrificial? Who needs that philosophy? All its gotten you, so far, is guilt. And that's all it ever will get you!"[3]

Here is explicit, straightforward, shall I call it moral instruction. The therapist in fact, later in this very first interview, goes on to deride the patient for attempting to be Jesus or Moses. This therapist is unique only in the sense that he is so clear about what he does. His theory is that people are sick because of their crazy beliefs, and among these are nonsensical moral obligations. The therapist reports that this patient dramatically improved as a result of the victory of rational self-interest over her insane moral obligations.

Now, I do not know whether this psychotherapist believes there are any sane moral obligations which are counter to rational self-interest. But it is clear that the essence of his psychological theory is that sanity is rational self-interest and his therapy is directed toward that goal.

The second possibility—that we have imported into our theories and our therapy our own moral attitudes and beliefs disguised as health values—continues to be a subject of enormous controversy in psychiatry today. I discussed that at length earlier.

But the question is, what shall we do about it now that we recognize the problems? Psychiatry is very much divided on this difficult matter. There are those who believe that we must acknowledge the truth of this argument and psychiatry should import some explicit vision of morality into its work. This belief, however, creates a struggle over what kind of morality that should be, and that has divided psychiatry into sects within schools. Do psychiatrists then have an obligation to reveal their moral values to patients in advance? This is not just a bizarre example of pushing an argument to an extreme. There are now, for example, radical psychiatrists, gay psychiatrists, Christian born-again psychiatrists, feminist psychiatrists, and other examples of an explicit conjunction of psychiatry and some specific value orientation, moral or ideological system. It cannot have escaped you that each of these conjunctions will generate not only different therapeutic objec- tives but different conceptions of mental disorder and its cure.

There are other psychiatrists, however, who are attempting to identify and remove the moral values from psychiatric theory and therapy. This purging of hidden morality has led to intense debate over which of the "health values" are "moral values." This is what happened in the case of the diagnosis of homosexuality, which I shall discuss in the next chapter. Here it should be noted that the decision that homosexual- ity per se was not a disease or a disorder was an extraordinary confession of our own uncertainty about the human condition and what salient aspects need to be explained.[4]

The third alternative, of respecting the patient's own values and moral convictions and working within that framework, is what most psychiatrists would want to claim they do. The practical importance of this argument for the psychiatrist is that it implies that we are all able to treat patients whose values and moral convictions are antithetical to our own. I have been enormously impressed by the ability of some psychia- trists to do just this and to feel compassion not only for patients whose values and moral convictions are antithetical to their own, but also for patients who morally are terrible people by all conventional standards: drug pushers, rapists, child molesters, arsonists, etc. But one of the secrets of this therapeutic compassion is that the psychiatrist believes these patients are sick, and that successful treatment will reduce the patient's immoral behavior and alter his values. Therapeutic compassion is not necessarily forgiving, but it is premised on the psychiatrist's ability to believe that immorality is psychopathological.

Many psychiatrists, I think, actually do believe this. There is a tendency for such psychiatrists to call every immoral act "acting out," implying that it is sick rather than bad. Many of these moral difficulties fade into the background when the psychiatrist stops being a concerned psychotherapist, ignores the patient's situation in life, and simply prescribes drugs. The psychiatrist need not even share the language of his patient. That situation has prevailed in many of our public state hospitals.

This, I believe, is part of the great current attractiveness of biological psychiatry. Not only is there a claim of greater effectiveness, but also the hasty retreat to explaining all psychopathology in terms of brain enzymes seems to promise an escape from the terrible moral dilemmas and entanglements which I have been rehearsing. "Scientific Psychiatry" wants to become the study of the organism, not of the person.

We have begun under this influence to reorder our conception of the categories of mental disorder so that they comport with our biological discoveries about the organism. It may well be that this is good and sensible; it is after all the way "normal" science progresses. It may be that psychosis should not be regarded as a life experience but rather as a dangerous medical illness of the organism for which there is a rapid, safe, and usually effective chemical treatment. But suppose the biological psychiatrist were to discover that parents whose children have died produce the identical chemical disturbances in their bloodstream that psychotically depressed persons do. Will we then conclude that these grieving parents are experiencing a *dangerous medical illness*? Will we believe it is appropriate to give them rapid, safe, and usually effective chemical treatment so that we can eradicate their biological depression? Or will we want to assert our own nonbiological ideas about what it means to be human? Does such science not begin to offend our most important intuitions about human nature?

PSYCHIATRISTS AS ARBITERS OF MORAL PROBLEMS

If the descriptions I have given you are correct, if psychiatry is really so confused about moral questions, then how is it that society for so long allowed us to be the arbiters of difficult moral problems? The answer I believe is that our moral ambiguity and confusion, our inability to frame hard moral questions, has been our greatest asset as society's decision makers.

Whenever there are hard moral conflicts to be resolved, it is socially and politically convenient to have a group of professionals who can redefine some of the toughest cases in a way that allows us to avoid paying the full price of our principles.

Consider the difficult moral questions attendant on abortion. Ten years ago the law in most states allowed abortion only when necessary to save the life of the pregnant woman or to preserve her health.[5] As public pressure began to mount against these strict legal restraints, the debate which we now know as freedom of choice versus right to life began. Early on, however, psychiatrists increasingly began to take advantage of the exception to the strict rule—that is, necessary to preserve the health or save the life of the woman. They resolved the difficult moral question in individual cases by invoking the nonmoral question—the mental health of the pregnant woman. The typical situation went like this: the woman who was desperate to have an abortion would be described by the sympathetic psychiatrist as "depressed and suicidal." The abortion therefore was necessary to keep the woman from putting her own life in danger. Since psychiatrists in effect controlled the only available access to safe legal abortions, you can imagine that many women who wanted abortions would have felt their only option was to simulate or exaggerate these sorts of symptoms. I was one of a group of psychiatrists who were called together to try and step back and look at what psychiatry was doing. Whatever therapeutic justification there may have been for psychiatric abortion, the data we assembled demonstrated that with psychiatrists controlling the abortion decision, middle- and upper-class women were twenty times more likely to receive a therapeutic abortion than lower-class women. And, we found that women dying after illegal abortion tended to be poor and black or Hispanic. We concluded, among other things, that with psychiatrists controlling the scarce resource of therapeutic abortions, it worked in a race- and class-biased fashion.[6]

An equally powerful example of this same unfairness occurred during the Vietnam war, when suddenly it seemed that, contrary to all previous demographic evidence, psychiatric illness was more prevalent among the middle and upper classes than among the lower class. At least this was the case among young men excused from military service because of psychiatric illness.

The abortion and Vietnam examples are, in my experience, typical. The psychiatrist, in the privacy of his office, in sympathy with his patient, renders a therapeutic solution of a moral problem. These decisions, when aggregated, reveal a discriminatory distribution of psychiatric mercy. This happens even when psychiatrists are neither just plain dishonest nor just partisan in their decisions. When we look closely, we see that our notion of fairness is twice cheated: moral principles are bent and they are bent in an inequitable fashion.

Sometimes people who hear my ideas on these topics tell me they think I have quite given up on psychiatry. I can assure you I have not. I cling to Hegel's aphorism that the owl of Minerva only spreads her wings at dusk. I admit, however, that it is well past nightfall and my continuing faith in psychiatry comes not from theoretical speculation, but from my experience as a psychotherapist. What follows is a description of a patient I have treated for 20 years. It will demonstrate at least that even psychiatrists deeply influenced by Freud's vision have some faith, hope, and charity. But I also believe that this case will help me to explore with you how I think and feel about psychiatry and morality in the face of all the confusion I have described.

A CASE EXAMPLE

Immanuel Kant, at the conclusion of *Anthropology from a Pragmatic Point of View*, described a kind of thought experiment as follows:

> It could be that on another planet there might be rational beings who could not think in any other way but aloud. These beings would not be able to have thoughts without voicing them at the same time . . . unless they are all as pure as angels, we cannot conceive how [these beings] would be able to live at peace with each other, how anyone could have any respect for anyone else, and how they could get along with each other.[7]

Now it turns out that Kant's imaginary beings of another planet exist in a certain way here on earth in the form of persons whom we psychiatrists describe as having schizophrenic disorder. It is not an uncommon symptom of such patients that they believe everyone else can read their minds. Thus, although there is no reciprocity in this mind reading, they suffer in some of the ways that Kant imagined.

I have treated one such patient, as I have said, for 20 years. She struggled to keep her mind as pure as an angel but, being human, she often failed, and would experience terrible feelings of shame and humiliation when people read her mind. These experiences entirely disrupted her life. She felt vulnerable, intruded upon, and defenseless. As Kant correctly predicted, she felt no one could have any respect for her. She twice had made serious suicide attempts. She was thought to be a hopeless, process schizophrenic. When she began treatment with me, she had constant auditory hallucinations and many complicated delu-sions, had twice been hospitalized in catatonic episodes, and had no sustained benefit from extensive electroconvulsive treatments. I cannot detail the many years of psychoanalytic therapy which spanned the era before and after the development of appropriate drug treatment. When I began treating her, she quickly formed the kind of intense attachment psychiatrists call a psychotic transference. She was obsessed with her great love for me, or as I repeatedly told her, her great love for her mother whom she had rediscovered in me. All of her hallucinations and delusions rapidly disappeared. The only loss of reality on her part was her conviction that I was equally in love with her, but temporarily unable to admit it. Five years of disordered schizophrenic thought cured by falling in love with her psychiatrist.

I cannot provide the details of her long and difficult treatment. But I can say that her feeling of being in love changed to loving, and out of her life story we constructed a new self-description relevant to her one persistent delusion—it has lasted 20 years—that her mind was being read. At some level of consciousness, she had never abandoned her mother's project for her; unconsciously it was her desire to be a star in the spotlight. At the same time, she was and is an extraordinarily vulnerable person. Measured against this project, her life was a failure, and she struggled against feelings of total inadequacy. Every social encounter was for her, at some level, a failed public appearance in which the spotlight was meant to be on her. It was from this perspective that I interpreted her delusion that her mind was being read by everyone in a rather standard way, as the pathological fulfillment of a fear and a wish: the fear that everyone would see her inadequacies and the wish that everyone would notice her—all this magnified by her vulnerability. The delusion that her mind was being read served to place a kind of spotlight on her. It was also a dramatic elaboration of her feelings of vulnerability. This new self-description allowed my patient to cope with what was both a feeling and a belief that her mind was being read. During therapy she began to realize that this feeling/belief came on in two kinds of situations, at times of particularly low esteem when she was isolated, lost and ignored in a social group, or in situations when others were in the spotlight and she was part of an anonymous crowd (for example, at the theater). When she became very disturbed, she would have the feeling/belief that the famous people she watched on television were reading her mind and speaking directly to her. The nature of these situations, I suggested, were confirming evidence for the fear/wish interpretation I had given her.

There are many aspects of this highly condensed example that one might discuss. Did we discover the truth about her life or did I merely indoctrinate her with one set of self-descriptions which have little or nothing to do with either her actual life or her delusion? And, even if these were in some sense correct self-descriptions, are they an example of the logical fallacy of assuming that *understanding* her memories about the history of her life and her desires is the same as *explaining* her delusion as though psychosis could be explained at the level of experience? Many psychiatrists today would consider this lengthy treatment process an absurd relic of a misguided era in psychiatry. They would attribute the relief of her symptoms to the drugs she was eventually given: a chemical imbalance in her brain no doubt explains her illness, and the drugs corrected that imbalance and explain the cure. Understanding her life, they would argue, is a different enterprise than explaining her psychotic disorder.

I have no hard scientific rejoinder to these biological claims, but if her schizophrenia was only a biochemical imbalance, how is it that falling in love with me was sufficient to cure all of her psychotic symptoms but one? Falling in love had in fact temporarily transformed this disordered, distracted, hallucinating woman. I want to consider this question of my patient's love and her mind-reading delusion. Although my patient said she believed and understood the fear/wish self-description she had worked out with me, periodically her faith would weaken. She would come back to me for—what shall we call it?—love, reassurance, reinforcement, or reindoctrination.

At these sessions I would ask her how after all these years, two decades, could she still believe that her mind was being read. She never has been able to explain either to her own satisfaction or to mine why she periodically relives Kant's thought experiment, but one thing is clear to both of us: that she gets something from the human relationship when she sees me that is temporarily sufficient to overcome the delusional belief and renew her faith in the therapeutic self-descriptions, sometimes for as long as three months. Now some people may feel this therapy is merely a form of conditioning, a positive reinforcement, and it may be. My own understanding is that her mind-reading delusion is a passionate conviction about her vulnerable situation in the world. Her delusion begins when she feels her self disappearing from other people's awareness. It requires both her understanding of what is happening and her sense of attachment to me to control this disappearance of self into vulnerability. In her case at least, it is not enough to keep the interpretation of all this vividly in the forefront of her consciousness.

She must also have a continuing sense of a loving connection with me, a sense that she exists in my awareness and I in hers.

LOVE, INSIGHT, AND CURE

Some of the description I have given is, I think, a commonplace experience for psychiatrists; it is the frustrating recognition that insight in the form of a new self-understanding is for many of our patients insufficient; they internalize the new self understanding only as they idealize the therapist. The supposed goal of orthodox psychoanalysis was to work through this idealization of the analyst, but this goal is seldom fully attained in my opinion. What studies there have been of patients who have been analyzed suggest that their failure to work through the idealized transference is a common occurrence. Enjoying this idealized transference is the secret vice of psychoanalysts. Even psychoanalysts themselves talk about their own psychoanalysts with a tone of reverence, or at least appreciation, which they rarely accord to mere mortals. But it may well be, as the example of my patient suggests, that these reverential feelings are in some way essential to the "cure" and to the stability of their new self-understanding.

We have reached the classic question: does psychotherapy cure by love or by insight? I would claim there is an analogous question: does moral conviction come from loving the moral instructor or from the wisdom of his teachings? The answer seems to me clear: both are involved in each case.

I shall talk only about psychotherapy. I will leave it to the moral philosophers to decide if there is, in fact, any parallel. Psychiatrists are accustomed to think of disorders of consciousness in terms of the traditional distinction between thoughts and feelings. There are thought disorders and mood disorders. There are irrational ideas and unnatural impulses. This dualism between cognition and affect is reflected in the notion of the struggle between reason and passion. Even our legal test of insanity reflects this dualism. There is on the one hand insanity manifested by the inability to *know* right from wrong, and there is insanity manifested by an irresistible *impulse*. But delusion is not just a false belief about the world; it is a passionate conviction. A phobia is not just a feeling of anxiety; it is also a false belief. Depression is not just a disorder of mood; self-loathing expresses a set of deep convictions about the self.

All mental disorders are in some sense passionate convictions about the situation of the self in the world. They are not just false beliefs; they are not just peculiar feelings. Mental disorder is a passion in the different sense that Roberto Unger has given it. Passion exists at the point "where distinctions between desire (wanting something from the other person) and knowledge (viewing him and myself in a certain way) collapse."[8]

Our patients, and I do not mean just our psychotic patients, seem reluctant or perhaps even unable to give up their passions. Passion is not so easily routed even by making the unconscious conscious. What I am trying to say by way of these arguments is that our most important convictions about ourselves and our situation in the world are passionate convictions, convictions which will change only when passion finds a new configuration. How does that happen in psychotherapy? First, consider therapy not performed by psychiatrists. My profession has for a long time recognized that alcoholics are better treated by Alcoholics Anonymous than by psychotherapy. Furthermore, it is clear that Alcoholics Anonymous affords both powerful attachments to a new group as well as moral instruction about one's situation in the world. The dramatically cured alcoholic is often a fanatic. The same is often the case with cured addicts. And, of course, similar things happen in cults. There is a powerful attachment to a new group and a profound change in one's convictions about oneself and one's situation in the world. Many of these "cures" are achieved with some better understanding of one's past (at least there is a confessional element), but a new and passionate conviction about the situation of the self in the world seems to be a crucial element of change.

You will recognize that in the view I am suggesting there is a considerable overlap between religious conversion and what goes on in the psychotherapist's office. The transference involves both a kind of love and the acceptance of the therapist as an authority about the subject of the situation of the self in the world. At the same time, the kind of intense transference or love that I described in my patient constituted in itself a new and passionate conviction about her situation in the world. Love, after all, is a profound change in one's experience of the self and its situation in the world. Love is perhaps the most powerful example we know of an experience at the point where the distinction be-tween desiring and knowing collapses. It is love—which, after all, is a passion—that suggests there is something wrong with the notion that life is a struggle between reason and passion. Love is such a powerful counterexample that it demands that we reconsider the traditional dichotomy. If delusions like love are, in fact, located at this point where the distinction between knowing and desiring collapses, perhaps that is why patients are not fully persuaded by psychological interpretations of how they come by their delusions and are not easily deprived of their idealized transference. This is not to say that psychological accounts like those I gave to my patient are without power. I believe that ideas have power to change people's lives, not just because reason can overcome inclination, but also because ideas can sometimes rally the passions.

If it is true, as it seems to be for many patients, that they rarely succeed in the task orthodox psychoanalysis sets for them of working through their idealization of their psychiatrists, then the enterprise of psychotherapy takes on a different aspect.

The crucial consideration is the psychiatrist as a person, his moral character, the kind of an ideal he presents to his patient. In the end, the most important thing about a psychiatrist is probably the kind of person he is and the kind of relationship he establishes. The psychoanalyst goes to great lengths to conceal the kind of person he is and to deny the reality of the relationship. But at some point he must speak and respond, and what he reveals about himself in those moments is more important than he has been taught to believe. And it may be that a cure is a moral achievement for the patient as well as the therapist. The patient achieves a new moral conviction about the situation of the self in the world. The therapist's achievement is to have given moral guidance without being a moralist.

The goal of self-fulfillment, the feeling of self-loathing, and the experience of loneliness: this is the neurotic syndrome of our time. Love and moral ambition seem to be the cure, but to many this sounds like a prescription to embrace vulnerability. They are trapped by the subjective experience that hostility and contempt seem to be what hold the self together. This inner toughness is the only security they know, and love and moral ambition threaten that security.

Here on the inner stage of the psyche is played out the same drama we see in the world. Perhaps this is only rhetorical analogy, but in both cases it seems that the fear of vulnerability becomes the enemy of life. In saying this, I risk making the error that Freud made of claiming to know the truth behind self-deception, of offering a prescriptive theory of the human condition. But the reader will have realized by now that I believe there is no alternative; the risk cannot be avoided. The therapist who has no vision of what it means to be human forfeits his own humanity and has none to offer the patient.

REFERENCES

1. K. Horney, *The Collected Works* (Norton, 1963).

2. P. Rieff, *Freud: The Mind of the Moralist* (Viking Press, 1959).

3. A. Ellis, *Growth Through Reason: Verbatim Cases in Rational-Emotive Therapy* (Science and Behavior Books, 1971), p. 228.

4. Stone, Presidential Address: Conceptual Ambiguity and Morality in Modern Psychiatry, *American Journal of Psychiatry*, Vol. 137, pp. 887–893 (1980).

5. For review of state abortion laws at that time, see *Report of the Task Force on Family Law and Policy to the Citizens Advisory Council on the Status of Women*, United States Department of Labor (Government Printing Office, 1968), pp. 28–29.

6. Committee on Psychiatry and Law, *Right to Abortion: A Psychiatric View*, Group for the Advancement of Psychiatry, Vol. VII, Report No. 75, October 1969.

7. Kant, *op. cit.*, p. 250.

8. R. M. Unger, A Program for Late Twentieth Century Psychiatry, *American Journal of Psychiatry*, Vol. 139, p. 159 (1982).

XI

Morality for Psychiatry

FREQUENTLY IN THESE ESSAYS reference has been made to the four competing paradigms of modern psychiatry. This analysis originated with Aaron Lazare, who described what he called the four "hidden conceptual models."[1] These models are today far from hidden: they have become the basis for the development of a kind of subspecialization within psychiatry. Although there are purists, almost all clinicians give some credence to all of the models in treatment. Lazare's example will allow me to recapitulate the models and what I have called the pragmatic eclectic approach.[2]

Lazare describes the schizophrenic patient who gets medication, which implies a biological etiology; who undergoes psychotherapy, which implies that past experience affects his present dysfunction; who is subject to a token economy, which implies that his behavior can be shaped by reinforcement; and who is a member of a therapeutic community, which implies that he should be reintegrated into a social system. What is a schizophrenic patient supposed to understand as the organizing theory behind all of what is being done to and for him? As Lazare points out, we psychiatrists have no comprehensive set of general laws that includes all the models—we have no unifying paradigm.

When we try to place bits and pieces of these models together, we cannot be sure that they really fit; they may, in fact, be orthogonal.

Psychiatry has these four competing paradigms—at least four "scientific" languages, and many dialects. There has been a tendency to exalt one model or the other as though it had all the correct answers. During the span of my own career the psychoanalytic, then the social, and now the biological have been in the ascendancy. (The behavioral model is also of increasing importance, particularly to other medical specialties such as pediatrics, internal medicine, and preventive medicine.) As biological psychiatry has come to the fore, there have been premature attempts to translate everything in human social reality into the language of neurosciences. The future of psychiatry may well belong to the neurosciences, but that time has not yet come. Mankind has not yet solved the mysteries of the mind, nor have the twentieth-century neuroscientists solved all of the mysteries of the brain. It may be exhilarating to translate everything that seems so subjective in psychiatry into a model that seems so objective. But surely humility is in order when things posited of the mind are forced into the language of the infant science of the brain.

It seemed to me that eclecticism as to theory and "pragmatic eclecticism" as to practice were preferable to this new biological reductionism. I therefore urged psychiatrists to practice diligent eclecticism and not forget our commitment to helping the whole person. Psychiatry, it seemed to me, was in danger of forgetting its humanistic commitment. I still believe that this is an important concern not just for psychiatry, but for all of medicine, which has moved in the direction of treating diseases rather than persons. However, partly because of my growing concern about the moral aspects of psychiatry, I became more aware of the problematic ambiguities of eclecticism in theory and in practice.

I therefore used the occasion of my Presidential Address to the American Psychiatric Association to discuss the conceptual and moral ambiguities of modern psychiatry.[3] I have made very minor changes in the "Address" because what I said on May 3, 1980, seems to me to present a moral challenge to psychiatry.

Last year in my response to the Presidential Address I rather presumptuously associated myself with the wisdom of the owl of Minerva—the owl that Hegel said only spreads its wings at dusk. From that lofty position I described a new era in psychiatry that I called pragmatic eclecticism, an era in which the four competing models in psychiatry had learned peaceful coexistence. These models—the biological, the psychodynamic, the behavioral, and the social—I suggested were held together by the medical model, which provided clinical coherence if not conceptual clarity. As I present the Presidential Address I must confess that the wings of the owl of Minerva were not fully extended last year. I recant nothing, but I now believe I glided too easily over that qualifying phrase about the absence of conceptual clarity. I intend to address the ambiguity of our eclecticism and my concern that having overcome the tyranny of narrow orthodoxy we are now in danger of retreating behind new walls. I shall touch briefly on subjects familiar to you all: racism, homosexuality, and the situation of women. I shall not attempt to deal with the substance of these matters; rather, my intention is to analyze how American psychiatry has grappled with them. These are all issues which have confronted psychiatrists in their practice, challenged the moral assumptions that lie concealed in our theories, and confounded us with disputes and acrimony in our Association. It is as we attempt to deal with this kind of issue that the new walls are being built, and it is no accident that each invites psychiatry to take a stand on human values. Human values, after all, are a crucial link in the chain that binds the self to society. To take a stand on them reveals something about our own selves, our own relation to society, and our own vision of what it means "to love and to work."

Many psychiatrists believe that our Association should limit itself to issues that are clearly psychiatric, and they look back at some of the strong positions we have taken on what they consider social issues with regret. Many other psychiatrists believe these social issues are clearly psychiatric; they are proud of what we have done and urge us to do more. I shall claim that what separates these two groups can only be understood as part of the deeper theoretical dilemma in which American psychiatry finds itself, its lack of conceptual clarity. I know I shall be addressing a subject in public which most of us prefer to talk about in private, but my temerity is sustained by three considerations. First, our professional training obliges us to understand conflict rather than to repress or deny it, and I believe that in view of recent events the time has come to confront this conflict openly. Second, I have become convinced that the basic limitation of pragmatic eclecticism is that it creates and sustains a mood of caution and expediency in all things, including matters that require moral ambition. Thus, perhaps without thinking it through, we are losing the courage of conscience. Finally, I do not intend to suggest an ultimate solution. I mean only to describe the problem as I encounter it in my own heart and mind.

THE PARABLE OF THE BLACK SERGEANT

I turn to what I have called the parable of the black sergeant. It is a parable about racism, about guilt and forgiveness, and about psychiatric
theory and practice. The identifying information in this parable/case
history have been disguised for reasons of confidentiality, but the value
conflicts it presents are real enough. The patient, a black man, was a
supply sergeant. He was caught by the military police stealing a
deodorant stick from the post exchange. The Army, which had reason
to suspect the sergeant of other thefts and was undeterred by constitutional restraints on search and seizure, went to his home and reclaimed
every piece of Army property which the sergeant could not account for.
The pile of supplies—uniforms, blankets, picks and shovels, cartons of
canned goods, mess kits, etc.—could have filled a trailer truck. It had all
been photographed on the sergeant's front lawn, and that picture
became part of his Army medical file.

The Army was determined to court-martial the sergeant, but he
had been examined by a civilian psychiatrist who decided that much of
what was stolen was of no use to the sergeant and, based on his
understanding of the sergeant's psychodynamics, had diagnosed him as
kleptomaniac. This civilian psychiatrist was prepared to testify at a
court-martial that the stealing was due to unconscious and irresistable
impulses. Unhappy with the civilian psychiatrist's report, the Army
sent the sergeant to be evaluated at an Army hospital. There he was told
repeatedly that anything he said could be used against him at the court-
martial. The sergeant took the warning rather impassively, and his Army
psychiatrist set to work to construct a very detailed anamnesis over the
course of three weeks.

The sergeant, who was a very intelligent man, got caught up in
telling the story of his life. He had grown up in a Southern city during
the days of racial segregation. A good and serious student from a deeply
religious family, he had done well in school and had gone to a small
college where he studied literature. After graduation, despite his hopes
and dreams, he had found no appropriate work and eventually was
drafted into the Korean War. After the war, seeing no alternatives, he
remained in the Army to serve his twenty years. As the years passed he
became increasingly bitter. He was convinced that life had cheated him
because he was black, and that the Army, in the work and in the
position it gave him, continued to discriminate against him. Out of this
sense of being cheated there grew a sense of entitlement, and he came to

feel that he was justified in taking whatever he could whenever he could. He had no sense of being impulsively driven to steal Army property; instead, he stole with a sense of entitlement and reparation in protest of the racist world that had deprived him of his hopes.

It is not clear why this black supply sergeant, despite being warned, told all this to the Army psychiatrist. At any rate he did, and the Army psychiatrist, after puzzling over the diagnostic possibilities (which included paranoid personality and depression), concluded that the sergeant did not have kleptomania or any other mental disorder which should excuse him from responsibility. Subsequently the Army psychiatrist testified at the court-martial. He told the story I have told you while trying to avoid the sergeant's eyes. The sergeant sat there in his dress uniform with his medals, his wife, and their small children. He was sentenced to five years at hard labor. As you may have guessed, I was the Army psychiatrist, and I felt something terrible happened that day. Each time my mind takes me back to that occasion I have a sense of dismay that will not be dissipated.

THE INFLUENCE OF MORALITY AND HISTORY

It is tempting when one reflects on this parable of the black sergeant to conclude that it demonstrates no more than the abyss between the moral concerns of the law and the therapeutic concerns of psychiatry. But none of us, I trust, would claim that if a man like the sergeant came voluntarily seeking treatment his psychiatrist would at no point consider moral issues. And how could one treat such a man with no moral perspective and revealing no opinion about racism? Surely a psychiatrist treating the sergeant in the 1980s would approach his problems differently than our predecessors would have done in the 1940s. Psychiatry does not stand outside history or morality, but how do we decide which history and which morality to accept? Is it all a matter of individual choice? Certainly one cannot find the rules controlling which history or morality to accept clearly delineated in the major theories of our biological, psychodynamic, behavioral, and social paradigms. Psychiatrists are taught to avoid value judgments in their dealings with patients, but I do not believe I make a radical claim when I assert that history and morality are a presence in the therapist's office. The only question is, how do they get there?

Let me turn to a narrower question: what role do our practice and our theory play in the courtroom drama of guilt and forgiveness? The legal system, even the Army's legal system, was hesitant to assess guilt in the face of a diagnosis of kleptomania. That diagnosis and the account of human behavior which goes with it invoke the unconscious and the symbolic meaning of the theft. Those who sit in judgment are not asked to consider the sergeant's race and social identity. His behavior is presented in isolation from its historical and cultural context. His kleptomania is understood in the confines of a personality development that repeats a timeless sequence outside culture and history. The psychiatrist, applying this kind of theory, comprehends the sergeant's motives as nonutilitarian and not intended to offend the system. Such a man can be forgiven; his quarrel is not with us but with his introjects.

On the other hand, the account I gave takes the man as he experiences his life within a particular culture and history. His stealing is understood as part of his response to his predicament. It is his revenge against an unjust system. Such a man cannot be forgiven by our law, but if his judges are willing to condemn the racism of their society, they can lighten his sentence. And if psychiatry is willing to lend its authority to the condemnation of a racist society we might even help the judges to reach that lighter sentence. But the moral and historical perspective that might have led me in that direction was not a presence in my office when I examined the sergeant. If in some sense I betrayed the sergeant, and I believe I did, it was because of the historical and moral perspective I brought to the subject of racism and my conviction that psychiatry was "objective."

PSYCHODYNAMIC VERSUS SOCIAL CONSIDERATION

I have carefully distinguished the psychodynamic and the social accounts of the sergeant's behavior, not only because that is how the two psychiatrists presented them, but also to emphasize the radically different moral implications and consequences of the two accounts. There is an irony here that should be underscored. The theory that excludes history and morality has the power to exculpate without disturbing the status quo. Thus the psychiatrist's choice of theory becomes crucial. I shall return to this question of choice. Many of you must be impatient with what seems an artificial distinction because as eclectics, we are all accustomed to invoking both accounts. Indeed, the word "psychosocial" seems to have been invented to make this point. Most of us are prepared to believe there was probably some truth in both accounts of the sergeant's behavior and to insist that anyone who hopes to understand the sergeant must give weight to both, not to mention biological and behavioral factors which are missing from this twenty-year-old parable.

Here we touch on the greatest strength of eclecticism and its greatest weakness. Its strength lies in its openness to consider the complexity of the forces that touch our lives. The eclectic psychiatrist sees biological man, moved by dynamic passions and ideals, shaped by culture and shaping culture. The eclectic has the most comprehensive view of what Sartre called the "critical mirror which alone offers man his image." But still that image is only a reflection; even less than a reflection, it is a composite sketch pieced together from the accounts of different witnesses whose vision depends on different theoretical perspectives. It is not just the problem of getting a biological, a psychodynamic, a behavioral, and a social pschiatrist to agree among themselves. How does the individual eclectic psychiatrist who conscientiously considers all of these factors reach a judgment about their relative significance?

This is our greatest weakness. We do not know what weight to give each perspective's account. We can diligently catalogue the different accounts. We can artfully construct Venn diagrams to suggest the possible relationships of these accounts. We can in rare instances assert with confidence the primacy of a particular account. But most often we are condemned to the ultimate ambiguity which is the inevitable consequence of our eclecticism. This is not a problem to be resolved by mere numbers; we do not have a formula or a way of deciding how much something should count. We psychiatrists often say that behavior is overdetermined, but might it be that this concept of overdetermination conceals our very deepest confusion, our inability to order the different considerations? As clinicians, each of us treats the whole person, and each day we try to piece together the composite sketch. But we also have a pressing responsibility to ease human suffering. Compassion draws us inevitably to expedient remedies. As pragmatic eclectics, uncertain that we have put the pieces of the picture together correctly, we can never be confident that we can distinguish between the sick patient and the sick society.

Lacking that ability and given that it is easier to apply expedient remedies to sick patients than to sick societies, will we not inevitably be led by our clinical responsibilities to distort the composite sketch of the human condition? At the very least we should understand that we might seem to the outside world to be doing just that.

SENSIBILITY AT THE COST OF AMBIGUITY

Here is a second irony to be underscored: it was only when our
generation of psychiatrists had the courage to overcome the walls of
narrow orthodoxy that we confronted our greatest weakness. Only
within the narrow paradigms could we construct if not a causal account,
at least something close to it. When we ventured outside we purchased
sensibility at the cost of ambiguity. This theoretical ambiguity is at the
very core of the conflicts that confound us. When we testify in court,
when we formulate our diagnostic nosology, when we issue position
papers, indeed, whenever we attempt to act, we confront this ambiguity. It is no wonder, then, that many psychiatrists are now eager to go
back to their narrow paradigms, where they hope to capture the rigor of
conceptual clarity that comforts the scientist and to escape from the
complexity of human values which accompany a greater sensibility.

Biologists, psychoanalysts, and behaviorists can at least imagine
this alternative, but social psychiatrists have no place to hide, no way to
narrow their sensibilities. They have always stood outside the walls
urging their colleagues to broaden their horizons. It might even be
possible to describe social psychiatry as the fractious adolescent member
of the psychiatric family, disrupting the serenity of the household by
arguing about values, morality, and social justice the way all adolescents
do. Shall we now expel them? Even if we could, I think it is too late.
The broad sensibility they brought to psychiatry has opened eyes that
will not be closed.

What I have described thus far is an honest picture of my own
perplexity, if not of yours. First, I know that I do not abandon history,
morality, and human values when I enter my office, but I do not know
how I decide what to take in with me. I believe that most of you are in
the same position, and for reasons I shall come to shortly I am deeply suspicious of anyone who makes the contrary claim that history, morality,
and human values are all irrelevant to psychiatry. Second, I know that I
at least am aware of no rules of ordering the different paradigms and
their interactions. When I sat in judgment of the black sergeant, I
believed that the objective truth of the matter was to be decided by
choosing the particular paradigm which best fit the facts of the case.
Having chosen the correct paradigm, I applied the explanatory theory of
that paradigm and thus never experienced a lack of conceptual clarity. In
a sense the four paradigms provided me a framework of differential
diagnosis within which I proceeded rigorously, with the skill and

objectivity of a scientist. My recognition that the goal of enlightened eclectics like Adolph Meyer was not to choose but to reconcile came when I began to examine the moral consequences of my professional activity. Is it possible that our inability to reconcile our paradigms stands in the way of both our scientific and our moral progress?

Thus far I have drawn a picture in which most of psychiatry might seem to stand to one side on the crucial questions of morality and human values, with only social psychiatry on the other side demanding that we get involved in the real world. But during this century all of science has learned painfully and tragically that science is not remote. Every thinking person knows that the physicist's equations play a crucial role in the destiny of humanity. Psychiatry's role is also crucial, although its influence is much more subtle. One of the most remarkable develop-ments in this century is the speed with which the psychiatrist's theories of human nature move from the arcane jargon of our journals through the mass media and into the consciousness of our culture. Psychiatry has played no small part in the transformation of the mind of modern man. This transformation takes place outside our control; theories are bowd-lerized and sensationalized. Our drugs are prescribed and self-prescribed everywhere. Other treatment methods have also been co-opted and arrayed in the struggles of interpersonal politics. Young people make love after they make therapy. There is in all the affairs of daily living, public and private, the pervasive if subtle influence of our profession.

The most powerful aspect of psychiatry is its contribution to what it means to be a person. This is not under our control, nor can it be in a free society. But we do bear a certain responsibility, and one of the themes in that responsibility is the hidden values in the theories and therapies that originated with us and contribute to the shaping of contemporary consciousness.

The thrust of this analysis is to claim that even without social psychiatry we are not on the other side. We have been engaged in an en-terprise that involves concealed positions on human values, moral postures, and even politics. This claim comes not just from unfriendly critics, it comes from responsible colleagues. This is the indictment that confronts those psychiatrists who assert that their psychiatry has nothing to do with these things; although the indictment can be overdrawn and viciously expressed, the fundamental truth in it cannot be gainsaid. Therefore, given the power of our enterprise, whether we like it or not we are in some measure responsible for the influence of these hidden values. It is also important to remember that many of us have wanted to use psychiatry to influence the public to confront and even to treat the sick society through the media. It is not just a matter of aloof scientists being victimized by the vulgarity of the mass media.

HOMOSEXUALITY

One of the first great battlefields in the attack on psychiatry's hidden values was homosexuality. Psychiatrists had long assumed that as part of their humanistic tradition they had brought their scientific perspective to things that were once considered evil. Homosexuality became sick-ness rather than sin, and this perspective in this century was accepted not only by the secular masses but even by most religious authorities. However, gay liberation brought a different perspective. Their argu-ment was that our judgments about homosexuality as sickness contained hidden values, a limited vision of human sensuality and intimacy, the old morality under a new guise, and perhaps even our own phobic limita-tions. A campaign was undertaken to remove the diagnosis of homosex-uality from the nomenclature. Our Association, after considerable deliberation and not a little acrimony, accepted that perspective. Our Association went even further—it called for an end to legal discrimina-tion against homosexuality. Here I come to the heart of the matter—the relationship of our lack of conceptual clarity to the actions we take. Recall the analysis I have developed here. Each of the four paradigms in psychiatry inevitably had its own theories about homosexuality.

Biological explanations can be sought in the endocrine system, psychodynamic explanations in childhood experiences and the Oedipus complex. Behaviorists can find answers in the sexual gratification reinforcement schedule. The social psychiatrist has the only paradigm that directly addresses the basic issues raised by gay liberation. Imagine if you will the eclectic psychiatrist who accepts all four paradigms but does not know how to reconcile them. Imagine such a psychiatrist who uses the four paradigms as a kind of differential diagnosis. Might that psychiatrist not conclude that there were four different kinds of homosexuality and that only the kind described by social psychiatry had been removed from our diagnostic manual?

This analysis may seem far-fetched and bizarre to you, but let me emphasize the structure of my argument. If we have no overarching theory which organizes the theories of the four basic paradigms, those paradigms cannot be changed from the top down—at least not by the logic of a controlling theory. Thus it is possible to argue that for many psychiatrists no fundamental change in their basic approach had occurred. They could go on as before. Therefore, the struggle for those concerned about gay liberation had to continue at a second level, which has two directions.

First, would psychiatry invest more in the effort to influence the public perception of homosexuality? Second, would each of the paradigms undertake the necessary theoretical reformulations essential to a fundamental change? My analysis in no way is meant to demean the decisions our Association reached. Nor do I minimize the importance of what we did. It was not an empty gesture. But I believe the real significance of our actions once again was moral. We changed the moral element in our composite sketch of homosexuality. I understand it as an act of moral compassion producing a small change in public perception. That small change in the long run can have a powerful effect.

WOMEN'S ISSUES

Perhaps the most penetrating and convincing attack on the hidden and destructive values in psychiatry has related to the subject of women. Indeed, when one has the occasion to read the standard works in psychiatry written before 1970, it no longer seems appropriate to talk about hidden values. It is no wonder, then, that psychiatrists who are concerned about the quality of the composite sketch of women promulgated by their profession and assimilated into our culture should turn to this Association to rectify it. There was obviously a great deal to be rectified, but they confronted an enormous obstacle. There was no diagnosis of female that could be expunged from the diagnostic manual; thus there could be no obvious battlefield. The struggle had to begin at the second level. How far would our Association go in its efforts to rectify the public's perception of women, and how thoroughgoing would be the necessary changes in the theoretical structure of each of the paradigms?

Here I come to the last piece in the structure of my analysis of how American psychiatry deals with these issues—that is, the effect of our own psychology and our own historical situation. As far as I can see, the case against psychiatry as regards women is far more damaging, requires far more than a minor adjustment of our composite sketch, indeed compels each of us to reexamine not only our theories and therapy but also our own lives and relationships. One might even say that psychiatry has only recently discovered that the maxim "to love and to work" applies to women.

Is it possible that the issues raised concerning women cut deeper in American psychiatry than even racism and homosexuality? That the questions raised in connection with women touch our personal as well as our professional identity? There can be no new psychology of women that does not require a new psychology of men. That makes necessary a new conception of all our human values and all the paradigms of psychiatry. This challenge comes at a time when our profession is struggling—when we have trimmed our sails and yearn for the safety of calmer waters. It comes at a time when many would like to retreat to their narrow paradigm. It comes at a time when the spirit of pragmatic expedience dominates our profession, narrows our horizons, and saps our moral courage.

Most psychiatrists are not by temperament polemical or adversarial. We do not seek out moral controversy. Most of us spend our lives listening compassionately to people who are suffering, whose lives are disrupted by the demands of passion and by the pains of helplessness. We try to be nonjudgmental while we help them weave together the delicate fabric of personal strength that sustains love and intimacy. And we sustain ourselves by small triumphs and acts of private altruism. Our successes often go unnoticed and our failures loom large. Ours is a vulnerable profession, easy to attack and to belittle, but it is a noble profession because it is both a moral and a scientific enterprise.

When we move from the safety of our office to take action in the real world we usually are motivated by the same moral enterprise that guides us in our office: a mixture of compassion, understanding, art, and science. The world outside our office may seem increasingly treacherous. But that treacherous world is already inside our office, if only in microcosm, and our work can never be carried on in a moral and historical vacuum. If like Hercules we were to succeed in lifting our giant of a science from its earthly connections, if we were to cut away all the links that hold self to society, then psychiatry would become a corpse. We will make mistakes if we go forward, but doing nothing can be the worst mistake. What is required of us is moral ambition. Until our composite sketch becomes a true portrait of humanity we must live with our uncertainty; we will grope, we will struggle, and our compassion may be our only guide and comfort.

REFERENCES

1. Lazare, Hidden Conceptual Models in Clinical Psychiatry, *New England Journal of Medicine*, Vol. 288, p. 345 (1973).

2. Stone, Response to the Presidential Address, *American Journal of Psychiatry*, Vol. 136, p. 1020 (1979).

3. Stone, Presidential Address: Conceptual Ambiguity and Morality in Modern Psychiatry, *American Journal of Psychiatry*, Vol. 137, pp. 887–893 (1980).

Index